FORGING

A HISTORY OF NURSING IN CANADA

DIANA J. MANSELL RN, PHD

A THOMAS PRESS PUBLICATION

ANN ARBOR, MICHIGAN

(2003)

DEAR LIZ
WORKING WITH YOU HAS
HELPED ME APPRECIATE
WOMEN & NURSES
OLD

First Edition, 2004

Edited by Diana Lauber

Published by Thomas Press/Ann Arbor, MI USA/www.thomas-press.com

Library of Congress Control Number: 2003103616

ISBN: 0-9728283-0-3

COVER ILLUSTRATION: Mary Agnes Snively, Founder of the Canadian National Association of Trained Nurses (CNATN) (foreground), and Alice Girard, CNA President 1958-1960 (background).

Cover design by Jennifer Heffelfinger.

CONTENTS

Acknowledgments iii

Introduction 1

1. THE BIRTH OF CANADIAN NURSING: 1870-1914 19

2. WAR AND EPIDEMIC: 1914-1919 43

3. THE DILEMMA OF THE 1920S 65

4. WEATHERING THE ECONOMIC STORM: THE 1930S 101

5. SUPPLY, DEMAND, ECONOMICS AND
   PROFESSIONALISM: WORLD WAR II 141

6. NURSING IN POST-WAR CANADA 169

Conclusion 185

Afterword: Unions, Leaders and Politicians: 1960-2000 191

Appendix: Presidents and Leaders of the CNA 207

Suggestions for Further Reading 211

Index 215

ACKNOWLEDGMENTS

I would like to thank all of the nursing leaders both past and present for their commitment to the profession that I have grown to love and hate, often at the same time. My nursing career spans 40 years and began at the Ottawa Civic Hospital at a time when students wore black stockings for their first 2 years, we lived in residence, we were exploited for service, our behaviour was closely monitored, and we loved every minute of it.

This project began in 1987 when I asked a colleague in the Nursing Faculty at the University of Calgary (UofC), "How did we get into the mess we're in?" Dr. Nancy Grant responded saying, "You're the historian, why don't you do the research?" At that time, my academic background consisted of a BA (Religious Studies) and an MA (British Indian History). With some guidance from Nancy and Shirley Stinson, I developed a Pilot Project proposal for the Alberta Heritage Foundation for Nursing Research (AHFNR) and was successful. Upon completion of the Pilot, AHFNR awarded me a grant that gave me the opportunity to study Canadian nursing leaders between 1920 and 1950.

To undertake this task, I travelled across Canada to interview roughly sixty nurses who had retired from leadership positions, and created a valuable collection of videotaped dialogues. Initial findings helped me to draw tentative conclusions regarding their varying leadership styles, but I was unable to uncover exactly what these women were trying to achieve as they shouldered Canadian nursing from the nineteenth-century through to the mid-twentieth-century. I am grateful to Nancy and Shirley along with other nursing

iii

colleagues, such as Dr. Margaret Allemang, Dr. Lynn Kirkwood, Dr. Meryn Stuart, Dr. Judith Hibberd, and the Ottawa Civic Hospital's Class of '63 for their encouragement and support along the way.

Another wise nurse suggested I take my video collection and use it to study the history of Canadian nursing while I was enrolled in the Doctoral program in the UofC History Department. Luckily, Dr. Donovan Williams (my MA supervisor) supported me in this venture and recommended I conduct the work under the competent supervision of Dr. Doug Francis. Dr. Tony Rasporich joined Doug and together their wit, patience, and attention to detail brought me through a somewhat arduous journey. Thanks to these able historians and to colleagues like Dr. David Bright, who accompanied me through the doctoral program and without whose humour I would probably not have survived.

Since the completion of the dissertation, I have worked on the manuscript to make it user-friendly and added an afterword to pursue the modern leadership debate. With regard to this work, I would like to thank Dr. Carolee Pollock for her assistance in editing and re-editing, and for contributing to many high-level discussions about nursing and nursing education over the years.

A number of archives and archivists assisted me in collecting the research data across Canada and in the UK. These people are the quiet ones without whose help historians would be destitute. I extend much appreciation to those individuals at the Helen Mussallem Library, the National Archives of Canada, the University of Toronto, the Alberta Association of Registered Nurses, the Glenbow Museum, and the British Library.

I also must thank my mother, Helen Fischer-Morrison, who steeled herself to live until my doctoral convocation before succumbing to lung cancer. Despite her failing health, she was a pillar of support as I worked to overcome the academic obstacles familiar to all doctoral students. My children, Diana and Will

Lauber, often endured the 'back burner' as I moved through the process. Their encouragement, support, and love throughout the decades is truly appreciated.

Last, but far from least, I would like to take this opportunity to thank my vast and varied circle of friends, which includes students, motorcycle companions, Mennonite buddies, Calgary Habitat friends, friends connected to Correctional Services Canada, and my Golden Retriever, Mitra.

To everyone above and those I may have missed, a huge thank–you and to the reader, I take full responsibility for all errors and omissions that might be discovered in this text.

Gassho, Namaste, and Bismillah.

INTRODUCTION

The year 2000 marked the beginning of what was to be official professional status for nursing in Canada. Canadian nursing associations had agreed that starting this year the basic educational preparation for a registered nurse is a baccalaureate degree. This decision was made by the Canadian Nurses Association in 1982 and those individuals who made the decision could not foresee the changes in health care and related services that would take place in the 1990s.[1] Has the push for professionalization through education on the part of nursing leadership contributed to the crisis in nursing at the beginning of the twenty-first century? Was the strategy of nursing educators misguided? It is only through a careful examination of the evolution of nursing in Canada that questions such as these can be answered. This book is such an examination.

Why has it not been done before? Historians have written extensively about Canadian women over the last three decades, but nursing has not claimed a significant share of their attention. Some have attributed this to an unconscious misogynist bias even in the work of researchers into women's history topics – nursing is too much the typical work of women, undervalued by society and even by women's advocates.[2] Although nurses play a fundamental role in the delivery of health care services, they are often left out of relevant histories. For example, a history of hospitals in Canada allocates a mere ten pages to the topic of nursing.[3] Essay collections in the history of medicine do not include nursing.[4] This omission in the history of health care may not be unexpected but it is more surprising in women's history.[5]

1

The neglect of nursing history is even more intriguing given the fact that between 1930 and 1966, membership in the Canadian Nurses Association grew from 8,000 to 79,312.[6] This number has now grown to over 100,000 and represents a significant proportion of women in Canada's workforce.[7] The work of nurses has attracted some attention from labour historians, but these historians have examined nursing history from the perspective of the worker and working-class relationships rather than looking at nursing as a whole.[8] Nurses do not fit very well into the categories employed by labour historians, nor do they fit easily into religious history or into women's history frameworks.[9] Mary Kinnear, in her book on professional women in Manitoba, devotes a chapter to nursing. While professionalization is the theme around which she organizes her material in this chapter, she emphasizes the subordinate position nurses held within health care. Kinnear acknowledges the contradictory interpretations of nursing that exist but cannot escape from them herself. Her work, while limited in scope – a mere chapter – represents a significant beginning by Canadian historians to include nurses in women's history.

British and American historians, by contrast, have gone much farther. The focus of British historians of nursing has changed with each generation.[10] A 1993 conference in Nottingham, "Nursing, Women's History and the Politics of Social Welfare," represented a major step forward in that the analysis of politics, power, gender, class and ethnicity were added to the earlier approaches to nursing history of professionalization and biography. Nevertheless, many British historians continue to agree that it is necessary to "dissect the processes of professionalization in order to understand how it was that independence gave way to subservience, dependency and exploitation." This dissection is important, not only in exposing the power struggles of the past, but also to "point towards a future in which nursing professionalism equates with autonomy," they argue.[11]

Nursing history has also attracted considerable scholarly attention in the United States. There, too, professionalization has been central to many of the studies.[12] Barbara Melosh added the issue of conflict in her study of American nursing. She considers the culture of work to be the 'mainstream' of nursing and deems professionalism to be merely an 'aberration'. Conflict resulted from the clash between the apprenticeship culture of rank-and-file nurses and the professional ideology of nursing leaders. Melosh concluded that the combined experience of professional ideology and apprenticeship culture allowed nurses to establish themselves as a "labor aristocracy among women" in the male public world of work. She argued that "the experience of paid work changes women's lives, sometimes in ways that challenge and disrupt existing notions of the place of women."[13] Nurses took pride in their competence and professionalism in the context of their workplace.

Susan Reverby organized her history of nursing in the U.S. around the notion of caring. She emphasized that conflict in nursing had to be understood within the context of a larger struggle with physicians and hospital authorities. These external authorities sought to define nursing and thereby control nurses. As she notes, nursing always had to struggle for the power to define itself or control entry into practice. In this situation, conflict was inevitable, "as nurses with conflicting class positions and sensibilities clashed over the definition of nursing, a coherent strategy for change and the meaning of womanhood."[14] This conflict constrained nursing reform in the U.S.

While conflict may have existed in Canadian nursing, it was far more muted than in the U.S. Professionalization has been one of the major interests of the few researchers into Canadian nursing, with much attention given to leadership, education and the subordination of nurses.[15] Early nursing history research tended to provide detailed chronological narratives, focusing on noted nurses in the field or a particular school of nursing. Most of these assumed that nursing "advanced" as a profession. Little of this material has been published in book or article form, remaining inaccessible as unpublished dissertations and theses.[16]

Kathryn McPherson examines the development of nursing in terms of skilled work and uses sources related to Manitoba nursing in her dissertation entitled, "Skilled Service and Women's Work: Canadian Nursing 1920-1939." In this excellent case study, she treats nursing as skilled work and concludes that for many Canadian nurses:

> gender and class operated together to create a unique occupational identity which blended professional dedication to service, workplace pride in skilled caring and personal confidence in the potential for economic self-sufficiency.[17]

McPherson does not set out to examine the role played by Canadian social, political or economic factors. She does examine the structure and content of nurses' work, the workforce, and nursing organizations in order to reclaim the experience, attitudes and actions of rank-and-file nurses as they forged an identity that defended nurses in the workplace and society. For these nurses, their struggle to gain status was rooted in the content and structure of nursing care, not the pursuit of professionalism. McPherson expanded this work into Bedside Matters: The Transformation of Canadian Nursing, 1900-1990 in which she focuses on how class, gender, and ethnicity interacted to influence the historical conditions of nursing in Canada.[18]

Where McPherson focused on the rank-and-file, this book focuses on the nursing leadership, particularly those involved in education. This close-knit elite set in place the fundamental definition of nursing in Canada. They did so by controlling both the Canadian Nurses Association and the editorial chair of The Canadian Nurse, the premier and for many years, the only, professional journal for nurses in Canada. In short, they filled the key leadership positions in Canadian nursing.[19]

The pursuit of professionalism was the motivating factor behind the activities of those nursing leaders who brought English-Canadian nursing through the first half of the twentieth century.[20] They were responsible for transforming nursing from a spiritual vocation to a secular profession. They were assisted in this task by the rapid growth in, and perceived need for, hospitals and hospital-based medical care that translated into a need for nurses and nursing care. The contribution made by the Nightingale legacy in the latter half of the nineteenth-century was that Canadian society assessed the work of nursing to be appropriate employment for young ladies. Therefore, nursing appealed to many young women and by the close of the nineteenth-century, a number of strong leaders emerged and began to organize themselves and their group of nurses. As the leadership moved nursing toward professional status, the support they received from general duty nurses was often passive but support nonetheless. The evidence suggests that rank-and-file nurses were more pre-occupied with issues relevant to the practical side of nursing than professionalism and thus, had little incentive to become involved in the ideological pursuits of the nursing leaders. This passive support was frequently associated with the desire of nurses to fulfill all of the demands that the public made on them. On the positive side, however, their enthusiastic desire to meet all of society's expectations garnered considerable public support for nursing. This support was important as nursing moved along the path to professionalism. Progress, however, was not continuous and linear. The professional cause advanced furthest when nursing concerns meshed with societal concerns, thus uniting the aspirations of both groups.

Furthermore, as a result of these efforts, nurses gained a self-esteem and self-confidence that gave them the courage to stand up for themselves and their vision of nursing in the face of any opposition emanating from the medical profession. Therefore, rather than being subordinate and subservient,

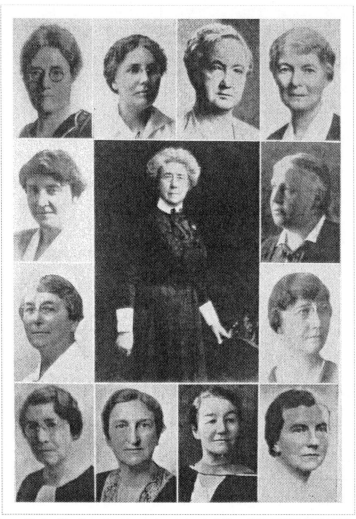

Early presidents of the Canadian Nurses Association, including: (CLOCKWISE FROM TOP LEFT) Mary Ard McKenzie 1912 - 14 / Scharley Wright Brown 1914 - 17 / Jean I Gunn 1917 - 20 / Edith MacPherson-Dickson 1920 - 22 / Jean E. Browne 1922 - 26 / (Centre) Mary Agnes Snively 1908 - 12 / Flora Madeleine Shaw 1926 - 27 / M. Hersey 1928 - 30 / Florence HM Emory 1930 - 34 / Ruby Simpson 1934 - 38 / Grace Fairley 1938 - 42 / Marion Lindeburgh OBE 1942 - 44 / Fanny Munroe 1944 - 46.

Canadian nurses actively pursued professional autonomy. Any success obtained by these women was due to their willingness to fulfill the nursing care needs of a Canadian society during a time of military, economic, or social crisis. In other words, nursing in Canada did not develop in a vacuum.

While some historians consider professionalism a limiting lens through which to examine nursing history, social scientists in other disciplines debate the concept from a much different perspective.[21] The sociological debate revolves around whether nursing is or is not a profession. Amitai Etzioni categorizes nursing among the semi-professions because nurses' training is shorter, their status is less legitimated, their right to privileged communication less established, there is less of a specialized body of knowledge, and they have less autonomy than "the" professions.[22] Fred Davis considers nursing to be a paradox as a profession because of its limited autonomy and authority, the small proportion of licensed nurses active in nursing, the relatively limited educational requirement and the growing chorus of complaint about the quality of nursing care from both health care professionals and the general public.[23] Eva Gamarnikow, however, focuses on nursing as a sexual division of labour subservient to the medical patriarchy: a subordination structure that comes to take on the ideological resonances of power relations between men and women.[24] By contrast, nursing authors such as Margaretta Styles, Reginald Pyne and Linda Hughes seem to be primarily concerned with the need to justify nursing as a profession.[25]

Mary Kinnear included nursing in her examination of professional women in Canada, and has argued her case convincingly.[26] Under her criteria for professionalism, Kinnear would include the following:

> postsecondary education and training in a subject requiring scientific or esoteric skill and knowledge; a certification test;

... a degree of self-regulation by practitioners ... [and] service to the public.[27]

In my examination of nursing, I have found that the term "professional" had different meanings at different times. It certainly included the aspirations that Kinnear mentions above at certain times, while at other times it took on a different meaning and emphasis. In essence, each generation of nursing leaders had its own vision of what was uppermost in the quest for professional status. My study highlights those ideals and changing visions from era to era. But underlying these multiple visions and aspirations lay one common thread: the need to believe that you were a professional. Nursing leaders were united in their desire to instil in nurses at all levels the belief that they were, or could become, professional. In order to be considered a professional by others, one must first believe that one is a professional. This was clearly the case for the nursing elite who are the subject of this study. Indeed, the word "profession" and the phrase "essential service" were used synonymously by these women to define nursing throughout the period covered. Although these women did not understand professionalism in the same way as it is understood and defined in current academic debates, their self-definition did, nevertheless, include many elements that we today consider to be criteria of "professionalism." It is the aim of this study to show what those criteria were and how their achievement moved nursing from a spiritual vocation to a secular profession.

The history of nursing is also important for understanding the experience of women's work in the past, and more importantly, for understanding health care, given that nurses' work occurred among the sick in a hospital or a home care setting. Sickness, as one of life's dominating threats, is a key experience for people. Furthermore, health care, medical interventions, and other related activities represent a juncture between private and public worlds.[28] The private and public world meet in the hospital setting that is "a special kind of community with its own individual character and traditions."[29] Given this unique setting for nursing activities, nursing became vulnerable to outside interference. Not surprisingly, therefore, a portion of its history was simply a reaction to pressure from outside.

Nurses participated actively in society and also in their own developmental progress. In fact, the history of nursing offers an example of women taking responsibility for shaping much of their future. Karl Marx stated that:

> men [and women] make their own history, but they do not make it just as they please; they do not make it under circumstances chosen by themselves, but under circumstances directly encountered, given and transmitted from the past.[30]

This was true for nursing in Canada as well. As nursing encountered the changing Canadian context, the profession transformed itself to meet new situations. This transition was not effected without difficulty. However, nurses themselves were responsible for the shift from nursing as a cooperative vocation to that of an indispensable profession.

Nursing did not develop in isolation; rather nursing participated in, and became very involved with, the lives of Canadians. As a result, much of the profession's development was in response to the needs of Canadian society, needs often identified by individuals and groups external to nursing. In the late nineteenth and early twentieth century, physicians who required low-priced staffing for their hospitals dictated these needs. During the First World War and the ensuing influenza epidemic, the role of the nurse was considered invaluable in the maintenance of the health of the Canadian public. Public health continued to be a concern until the outbreak of the Second World War at which point the government's demand for nurses to serve both at home and overseas placed incredible pressure on the resources of the profession. By the end of the War, nursing had risen in the estimation of many Canadians and had met the demands so successfully that the clamour for nursing service reached unanticipated levels.

Societal need definitely contributed to the changing nursing profession during this period, but desire for professionalism from within was a driving force as well. This is most obvious in the improvements made in nursing education. Nursing leaders worked tirelessly to move nursing education out from under the oppressive and dependent environment of the hospital into the independence of post-secondary institutions. The success that they realized contributed to a changing public perception of nursing. By 1945, many nurses were enrolled in universities across Canada acquiring post-graduate certificates in nursing specialties, further confirmation of the fact that nursing in Canada was no longer a spiritual vocation but a secular profession.

This transition occurred as well in terms of the image of the nurse. The 'good nurse' of the late-nineteenth century was expected to possess characteristics that identified her as a member of a spiritual vocation.[31] A promotional manual for nursing published in 1898 itemized these qualities:

Love of God and of fellow creatures.
Strength of body and mind.
Cheerfulness.
Belief that cleanliness is next to godliness.
Refinement of character.
Good education.
Knowledge of human nature.
Quickness of comprehension and action.
Patience and perseverance.[32]

By the close of the Second World War, the image of the 'good' nurse had undergone a radical transformation from that of 1898. In 1947, the editor-physician of the <u>Canadian Journal of Public Health</u> observed:

10

The nurse today holds a very enviable place in our society; every door is open to her; she has the respect and affection of all classes. She has gained this position in the last half century, not because she ever made it an objective, not because of her technical skill, or intellectual attainment, high though these are, not because of her ability 'to soothe the fevered brow'; almost surely she has attained her position through her indomitable will to serve, her readiness and capacity at all times and under all circumstances - from the hospital ward and the home to the forward surgical unit in war - to undertake and fulfill all the residual demands of the sick environment.[33]

Clearly, the role the nurse played during the Second World War contributed to this changed perception of nursing but the evolving hospital environment cannot be ignored.

What factors contributed to this change from vocation to profession? What role, if any, did nursing leaders or general duty nurses play? Have these changes benefited nursing, health care delivery, and Canadian society? If so, in what way and if not, why not? Furthermore, did society value the nurses' work? If the work was valued, how was it valued and by whom? Finally, in what way, if any, did medicine and Canadian society influence the developments in nursing? These questions will be answered as a result of a close examination of the history of nursing in Canada up to 1950.

Nursing will be analyzed through the experience of nursing leaders, the experience of the nurse working in the hospital, and to a lesser degree, the experience of the public health nurse. Finally, the role played by the public's perception of the nurse as expressed in popular culture will be included to complete the picture. The Canadian nursing experience will be placed within the political, economic, and social context of this period in order to develop a more comprehensive picture of Canadian nursing history.

A feminist perspective does not limit this discussion. Indeed, nurses and feminists have had a great deal of difficulty coming to any consensus on any topic and the debate has often revolved around ideas associated with "the feminist disdain for nursing."[34] The scorn felt by nurses is usually associated with their perception that feminists devalue the work of nurses. Feminists often portray nurses as subordinate to physicians because in their view, the medical profession "attains and maintains its position by virtue of the protection and patronage of some elite segment of society which has been persuaded there is special value in its work that discourages others and that requires others (like nurses) to be subordinated to the profession."[35] Was this subordination real or apparent? The group of nurses who are the focus of this study would deny that either individually or collectively, nursing was in any way subordinate to the medical profession.[36]

It is fundamentally important that the experience of these nurses be the basis for this particular history of nursing. It is important to pay attention to the fact that nurses, up to 1950, did, in fact, experience subordination, victimhood, and powerlessness but did not see it this way. They viewed their relationship with other health care providers i.e., medicine, as collaborative and equal. This group of women demonstrated proactive behaviour during a time period when many women responded to subjugation by remaining passive.[37]

Before examining the development of nursing in Canada perhaps it would be wise to define the term 'nurse'. It is not as simple as you might imagine. In the introduction to his book on the sociology of nursing, Fred Davis commented that in everyday speaking, the nouns "nurse" and "nursing" are applied:

> indiscriminately to a wide variety of health care activities, carried on in different settings, ... and to an occupation that includes some of the least-educated members of society

(such as aides and orderlies) and some of the most educated.[38]

In this book, we will trace the evolution of a definition of nursing which began to use registration and training as criteria for inclusion in the definition. But this did not occur until the 1920s. In the earlier period, any person who provided nursing care for pay would have been considered a nurse.

Given the contemporary importance of health care reform and its effect on services such as nursing, this analysis will bring clarification to an important area of health care services and women's studies in Canada. It will be shown that nursing was not always subordinate to the medical profession or that of the bureaucracy of the health care industry. Indeed, nursing was made up of women who brought credibility, legitimacy and professionalism to an aspect of women's work that historically had been undervalued by society. It is time to investigate the overall development of nursing in Canada in order to gain some understanding of how one group of women professionalized and brought credibility to a long-standing function that was expected of women: responsibility for maintaining family and community health.[39] It is their ultimate success in this undertaking that may have contributed to the gradual disappearance of nurses from the large urban medical centres of the 1990s. In these centres individuals classified as Licensed Practical Nurses, Certified Nursing Assistants, and Patient Care Attendants are replacing the professionally prepared nurse. These workers are far less costly than a professional nurse. Can this apparent demise of traditional nursing be attributed to the fact that "the pillars of secular nursing became humility, sacrifice, selflessness and obedience" or is it to be found in the successful attainment of professionalism?[40] An analysis such as this will contribute to an understanding of this conundrum and therefore add to the ongoing debate in Canadian nursing historiography.

NOTES TO INTRODUCTION

[1] Janet Kerr and Janetta MacPhail, <u>Canadian Nursing: Issues and Perspectives</u>, (Toronto: McGraw-Hill Ryerson Limited, 1988) p. 261. Also note that support from various provincial jurisdictions has not been forthcoming.

[2] Ellen Lewin and Virginia Oleson eds., <u>Women, Health and History</u>, (New York: Tavistock Publications, 1985), p. 9.

[3] G. Harvey Agnew, <u>Canadian Hospitals, 1920 to 1970: A Dramatic Half-Century</u>, (Toronto: University of Toronto Press, 1974), p.124. The author, a physician, closes his discussion of educational developments in nursing with the reminder that "the nurse must put the interests of her patients above her own."

[4] Wendy Mitchinson & J.D. McGinnis, eds., <u>Essays in the History of Canadian Medicine</u>, (Toronto: McClelland & Stewart, 1988); Charles G. Roland, ed., <u>Health, Disease and Medicine: Essays in Canadian History</u>, (Toronto: The Hannah Institute for the History of Medicine, 1984); and S.E.D. Shortt, <u>Medicine in Canadian Society</u>, (Montreal: McGill Queen's University Press, 1981).

[5] Nurses and nursing are given scant attention in Alison Prentice et al., <u>Canadian Women: A History</u> (Toronto: Harcourt Brace Jovanovich, 1986) and in Veronica Strong-Boag, <u>A New Day Recalled: Lives of Girls and Women in English Canada</u>, (Markham: Penguin, 1988). It should be noted that the situation is changing, albeit slowly see Dianne Dodd and Deborah Gorham, eds., <u>Caring and Curing: Historical Perspectives on Women and Healing in Canada</u>, (Ottawa: University of Ottawa Press, 1994).

[6] The Canadian Nurses Association, <u>The Leaf and the Lamp</u>, (Ottawa, Canadian Nurses Association, 1968), pp. 86, 96.

[7] This number does not include the many nurses in Ontario who are members of the College of Nurses of Ontario or nurses in Quebec.

[8] Kathryn McPherson, "Skilled Service and Women's Work: Canadian Nursing 1920-1939," Ph.D. Dissertation, Simon Fraser University, 1989; <u>Bedside Matters: The Transformation of Canadian Nursing</u>, 1900-1990, Toronto: Oxford University Press, 1996; David Coburn, "The Development of Canadian Nursing: Professionalization and

Proletarianization," International Journal of Health Services, Vol. 18, no. 3, 1988, pp. 437-456.

[9] Kathryn McPherson and Meryn Stuart, "Guest Editorial: Writing Nursing History in Canada," Canadian Bulletin of Medical History, Vol. 11, no.1, 1994.

[10] See Christopher Maggs, ed., Nursing History: State of the Art, (London: Croom Helm, 1987), p. 4; Rosemary White, Social Change & the Development of the Nursing Profession, (London: Henry Kimpton Publishers, 1978); Celia Davies, ed., Rewriting Nursing History, (London: Croom Helm, 1980); Anne Hudson Jones, Images of Nurses: Perspectives from History, Art, and Literature, (Philadelphia: University of Pennsylvania Press, 1988).

[11] Christopher Maggs, Nursing History, p. 5. See also, E. Smyth et al. eds., Challenging Professions: Historical and Contemporary Perspectives on Women's Professional Work. (Toronto: University of Toronto Press, 1999).

[12] Ellen Condliffe Lagemann, ed., Nursing History: New Perspectives, New Possibilities, (New York; Teachers College, 1983).

[13] Barbara Melosh, 'The Physician's Hand: Work Culture and Conflict in American Nursing, (Philadelphia: Temple University Press, 1982), pp. 6, 218-19.

[14] Susan Reverby, Ordered to Care: The Dilemma of American Nursing, 1857-1945, (London: Cambridge University Press, 1987), p. 200.

[15] See, in particular, the special issues of Canadian journals dedicated to nursing history, The Canadian Bulletin of Medical History, Vol. 11, no.1, 1994 and the Fall, 1995 issue of The Canadian Journal of Nursing Research, Vol. 27, no. 3.

[16] See Pauline Paul, "A History of the Edmonton General Hospital, 1895-1970, "Be Faithful to the Duties of Your Calling," Unpublished Ph.D. Dissertation, University of Alberta, 1994; M.E. Stuart, "Ideology and Experience: Public Health Nursing and the Ontario Rural Child Welfare Project," Unpublished Ph.D. Dissertation, University of Pennsylvania, 1989; Marie des Loyer, "Leadership and the Effectiveness of Community Health Nursing Services," Unpublished Ph.D. Dissertation, University of Ottawa, 1981; Georgette Desjean, "The Problem of Leadership in French Canadian Nursing," Unpublished Ph.D. Dissertation, Wayne State University, 1975; Linda B. McIntyre, "Towards a Redefinition of Status: Professionalism in Canadian Nursing 1939-1945," Unpublished M.A.

Thesis, University of Western Ontario, 1984; Phyllis Edith Jones, "The Family Physician and the Public Health Nurse: An Investigation of One Method of Collaboration," Unpublished M.Sc. Thesis, University of Toronto, 1969; M.J.Hoare, "Social Origins of Nurses and Career Satisfaction: A Study of Student Nurses in Three Metropolitan Halifax Schools of Nursing," Unpublished Master's Thesis, Dalhousie University, 1970.

[17] K. McPherson, "Skilled Service and Women's Work:...," Unpublished Ph.D. Dissertation, Simon Fraser University, 1989, p.411

[18] Kathryn McPherson, Bedside Matters:.... p.12.

[19] See Appendix for illustration of their close connections.

[20] It should be noted at the outset that this study deals with only the history of secular nursing in Canada. The experience of the Catholic nursing sisters was entirely different. In fact, it was often against that model that secular nursing leaders defined their profession. See Marta Danylewycz, Taking the Veil: An Alternative to Marriage, Motherhood, and Spinsterhood in Quebec, 1840-1920, (Toronto: McClelland and Stewart, 1987).

[21] See Jo Ann Whittaker, "Professionalization and Gender: The Case of the Registered Nurses of British Columbia," Unpublished Paper for the Fifth BC Studies Conference, November 4-5, 1988.

[22] Amitai Etzioni ed., The Semi-Professions and Their Organization, (New York: The Free Press, 1969), p. v.

[23] Fred Davis, The Nursing Profession: Five Sociological Essays, pp. vii,viii.

[24] Eva Gamarnikow, "Sexual Division of Labour: The Case of Nursing" in Annette Kuhn and Ann Marie Wolfe ed., Feminism and Materialism Women as Modes of Production, (London: Routledge and Kegan Paul, 1978), p. 97.

[25] Margaretta Styles, On Nursing: Toward A New Endowment, (St.Louis: Mosby, 1982); Reginald H. Pyne, Professional Discipline in Nursing, (Oxford: Blackwell Scientific Publications, 1981) and Linda Hughes, "Professionalizing Domesticity: A Synthesis of Selected Nursing Historiography," Advanced Nursing Science, 1990:12(4): 25-31. For a discussion of such changes in the context of the American medical profession, see E. Richard Brown, Rockefeller Medicine Men: Medicine and Capitalism in America, (Berkeley: University of California Press, 1979).

[26] Mary Kinnear, In Subordination, pp. 6-14.

[27] Ibid., p. 7.

[28] Roy Porter, Patients and Practitioners, (Cambridge: Cambridge University Press, 1985), p. 22.

[29] Noel Poynter, Medicine and Man, (London: C.A.Watts & Co.Ltd., 1971), p. 15.

[30] Quoted in E.P. Thompson, The Making of the English Working Class, (Harmonsworth: Penguin, 1963), p. 10.

[31] Although the term vocation has come to be almost interchangeable with occupation, it retains even today some of the odour of sanctity of its original meaning - a call from God. Nightingale understood nursing to be a spiritual calling. To a great extent, the move to professionalism is a renunciation of this understanding and its replacement by an equally lofty but secular ideal.

[32] Jane Hodson, How to Become a Trained Nurse: A Manual of Information, (New York, 1898), p. 11.

[33] "The Shortage of Nurses," CJPH, November, 1947, p. 549.

[34] Ellen D. Baer. "The Feminist Disdain for Nursing," The New York Times, February 23, 1991. This article was followed by Susan Reverby's discussion, "Other Tales of the Nursing-Feminism Connection," Nursing & Health Care, 14:6, June, 1993, pp.296-301. Also see Barbara Keddy, "The Coming of Age of Feminist Research in Canadian Nursing," Canadian Journal of Nursing Research, Summer, 1992, 24(2), pp.5-10. P.E.B. Valentine, "Feminism: A Four-Letter Word?," Canadian Nurse (CN), December 1992, p.20.

[35] Janice Acton et al. Women at Work Ontario 1850-1930. (Toronto: Women's Educational Press, 1974)

[36] See videotape collection of retired nurses in author's possession.

[37] This topic will be investigated through a variety of primary and secondary source materials. Primary sources include textbooks and articles written by leaders in the nursing profession. The records of the Canadian Nurses Association are examined as are The Canadian Nurse and other relevant journals in order to gain insight into the perspective held by nurses during this time period. Although from its inception in 1905 to the late-1940s, subscribers to The Canadian Nurse represented approximately thirty percent of the total number of registered nurses in Canada, all groups participated in topical debates through their particular clinical section of the journal. Public health nurses, private

duty nurses, nurse educators, and nursing leaders all had a section of the journal devoted to their concerns. The ideas expressed in The Canadian Nurse were those held by the nursing leaders in Canada. The overlap between the editorship of The Canadian Nurse, the presidents, and executive directors of the Canadian Nurses Association ensured that this was the case. The Appendix also shows that the presidents of the Canadian Nurses Association held positions of leadership throughout the country during their tenure of office. They defined nursing as a profession and their definition went largely unquestioned by the rank-and-file. In fact, they provided a self-definition that nurses could use. Medical progress that affected nursing will be tracked through primary sources such as The Lancet, Health and Home, and The Hospital and Nursing World. One final previously untapped primary source is data collected from an oral history project in which nurses who were active during this time period were interviewed on audiotape and videotape. Secondary sources will consist of the limited number of studies done on various aspects of nursing as well as histories of nursing schools in Canada.

[38] Fred Davis, ed., The Nursing Profession: Five Sociological Essays, (London: John Wiley & Sons, Inc., 1966), p. vii-viii.

[39] Strong-Boag, "Making a Difference," p. 239.

[40] Hilda Steppe, "Historical Research in Nursing" in 1990 Proceedings of the 5th Biennial Conference of the Workgroup of European Nurse Researchers, Collaborative Research and Its Implementation in Nursing, Vol.1, p. 308.

Chapter One

THE BIRTH OF CANADIAN NURSING: 1870-1914

The following poem entitled "The Nurse," was published in the first issue of <u>The Canadian Nurse</u> in March, 1905:

I lay my hand on your aching brow,
Softly so! And the pain grows still.
The moisture clings to my soothing palm,
And you sleep because I will.
You forget I am here? 'Tis the darkness hides.
I am always here, and your needs I know.
I tide you over the long, long night.
To the shores of the morning glow.

So God's hand touches the aching soul,
Softly so! And the pain grows still.
All grief and woe from the soul He draws,
And we rest because He wills.
We forget, - and yet He is always here!
He knows our needs and He heeds our sighs,
No night so long but He soothes and stills
Till the dawn-light rims the skies.[1]

This poem was not written specifically for <u>The Canadian Nurse</u> but the fact that it appears in the inaugural issue reflects the ideological foundation on which nursing was based after its first thirty years of existence.

Keeping in mind that <u>The Canadian Nurse</u> was the official organ of the newly emerging nursing profession; its views reflected those of the nursing leaders of the day. What this poem reflects in its reverential, romantic tone was the belief of the day that nursing was a spiritual vocation. This perspective grew out of the legacy of Florence Nightingale, the context of social reform, and the ambition of the medical profession.

The birth of Canadian nursing occurred in a nineteenth-century climate of medical advances and social reform. The advances made in medical science validated medical care thereby encouraging Canadians to look to physicians for solutions to their increasing health problems. In this way, Canadians, with their growing faith in reform, science, and physicians laid the groundwork for the eventual need they had for nursing service. In order to discharge their professional responsibilities, individual members of the medical profession built their own hospitals and established nursing schools attached to these hospitals in order to staff their institutions.

The vocational ideology was transferred from England where it was rooted in the Florence Nightingale tradition. The Nightingale ideology portrayed nursing as a spiritual vocation appropriate for the young ladies of Victorian society to pursue. Physicians imported the Nightingale system of education that positioned nursing under the directive eye of medicine but, at the same time, assured nursing of a role in the delivery of health care services. Although somewhat isolated from society behind the walls of the hospital and the nurses' home, this seclusion gave nurses the opportunity not only to acquire the necessary skills to care for the sick but also to develop a nursing culture within which they planned a professional future for nursing.

As the twentieth century dawned, nurses asserted themselves and began to take control of their destiny. Nursing leaders formed a national association and became involved on an international level with other nursing organizations. As in any successful birthing process, there existed a nurturing social environment in which all three components, nursing, medicine, and society, each had a need for each other, hence guaranteeing the survival of nursing into the twentieth-century.

The key to all of the developments in nursing that occurred during these early years was reform. The reforming ideas that shaped the changing nineteenth-century Canadian society evolved from an increasing faith in the power of science. Liberal Christians in Canada placed their faith in the leadership offered by the new social sciences, thus bringing together sacred and secular notions. According to historian Ramsay Cook, "advocates of the social gospel were in fact making the church irrelevant in a world where other institutions were better equipped to perform the socially useful roles once fulfilled by the church."[2] Consequently, the reforming spirit also transformed the popular view of both hospitals and nurses. The buildings that had previously housed the "sick-poor" became medical care institutions and the "Sairey Gamp" image of nursing that had been popularized by Charles Dickens became a respectable "lady-nurse."

This transformation occurred as a direct result of the enormous advances made in medical knowledge. By the 1830s, the microscope became widely available; ether was introduced in 1846; and the availability of chloroform followed soon after. The emergence of anesthetics allowed for more dramatic surgical interventions and this, in turn, shifted the location of treatment from the home to the hospital. These changes only added to the faith and confidence Canadians placed in the science of medicine. These advances in medical science contributed to the acceptance by Canadian society of hospital-delivered medical care.

This was also a time during which hygiene was a prevailing concern. Ideas associated with health and sanitation were discussed at length in the publication entitled Health and Home, self-described as "The official organ of the Canadian Sanitary

21

Association." The motto, boldly stated on the cover page, was "Pure Air, Pure Light, Wholesome Food and Cleanliness, Long Life, Manliness and Beauty." The journal published a monthly column entitled, "Care of the Sick." Its rationale for such a column ran as follows:

> To know how to take proper care of the sick is of the utmost importance to the attending physician who often loses a patient from neglect, or want of care, in nursing; and physicians will recognize with pleasure these suggestions, as to what should be done in case of accident to give relief, or to save life, until medical aid can be obtained.[3]

Consequently, the relationship between cleanliness and health was noted and eventually linked to the need for hospitals and health care. The increasing acceptance of hospital-care necessitated the construction of more health care institutions that would, in turn, require nursing staff.

The hospital of the day did not appeal, however, to the majority of the Canadian public. Early nineteenth-century hospitals were homes for the poor and the destitute and were staffed by individuals from a similar class. Therefore, the term 'nurse' bore no similarity to the more modern and evolved understanding of the term in the twentieth century. Given this context, nursing did not play a visible, or important role in the hospital. For example, nursing services were non-existent in the progress made by the Montreal General Hospital as outlined in the 1825 publication entitled, "An Account of the Origin, Rise and Progress of the Montreal General Hospital." The Montreal General had been established in 1820 "for the reception and cure of the diseased poor, and others who may not have the means or conveniency[sic] of being duly cared for when sick, at their own places of residence."[4] In spite of the fact that this mission statement would appear to involve nursing care, the word "nurse" appeared only once in the twenty-eight page narrative. Indeed, the situation was such that hospital funds were taken to purchase

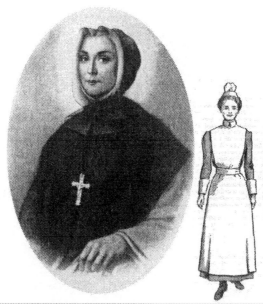

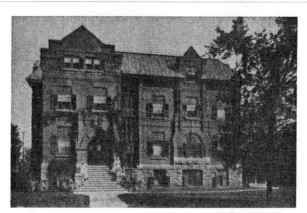

CLOCKWISE FROM TOP LEFT: Marguerite D'Youville, founder of the Sisters of Charity of Montreal, "Grey Nuns." (Courtesy Sisters of Charity) / Late nineteenth-century student nurse in the uniform of Vancouver General Hospital's School of Nursing. (Courtesy Vancouver General Alumnae) / Lady Stanley Institute, the first training school for nurses in Ottawa (Courtesy Ottawa Civic Hospital Alumnae).

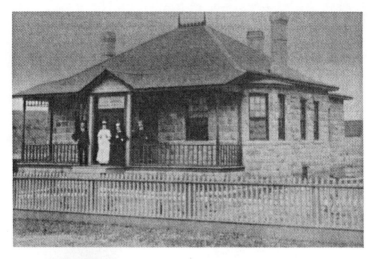

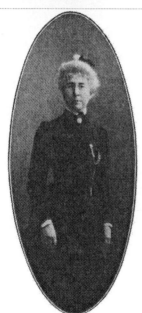

TOP: A maternity hospital in Medicine Hat. Medicine Hat was the capitol of what was then the Northwest Territories.

LEFT: Mary Agnes Snively, Founder of the Canadian National Association of Trained Nurses (CNATN). (Courtesy Toronto General Hospital Alumnae)

champagne and nurses slept in cubicles festooned with snow after a stormy night.[5]

It would appear that there was good reason for a derogatory view of nursing. An early nineteenth-century physician described nurses at the Montreal General Hospital as follows:

> Age and frowsiness seemed to be the chief attributes of the nurse, who was ill-educated and was often made more unattractive by the vinous odor of her breath. Cleanliness was not a feature of the nurse, ward or the patient; the language was frequently painful and free ... Armies of rats frequently disported themselves about the wards and picked up scraps left by the patients and sometimes attacked the patients themselves.[6]

In spite of these negative observations, nursing came to be viewed as a necessary part of progressive medical interventions. In his address delivered to the Canadian Medical Association in 1873, Sir James Alexander Grant stated:

> There is a point to which I would now desire to call the attention of this Association, viz., the advisability of having thoroughly trained female nurses. In private as well as hospital practice we constantly experience a great want in this respect. In each of the large cities having extensive hospital accommodation, some system might be inaugurated by which those desirous of becoming skilled nurses might avail themselves of the facilities offered, and in course of time, supply a deficiency now generally felt in the practice of the profession.[7]

But in order to make the work of the nurse acceptable to late-Victorian society, changes had to be made to the prevailing view of nursing.

The ideas of Florence Nightingale, first introduced in Canada in the 1870s, provided the solution to this dilemma and effected considerable changes in nursing. Furthermore, her legacy had a direct and significant impact on later developments in the profession. Nightingale viewed herself as a broadly based social reformer. Indeed, she believed that, "the specific business of nursing was 'the least important of the functions into which she had been forced'."[8] Nevertheless, she did see nursing as one means of achieving the perfect Christian society. Her determined efforts have gained her the reputation of being the founder of modern nursing.

The Crimean War gave Nightingale a perfect opportunity to set the tone for nursing. In the "Memorandum of Agreement" that she insisted all nurses who accompanied her to the Crimea sign, she set out her perspective on nursing. In the agreement, Nightingale agreed to employ the nurse to care for the sick and wounded members of the British Army and in return she would provide a salary, cover all travel expenses and provide board and lodging. The contract was negated if the nurse did not fulfill her responsibilities which involved devotion to duty, moral conduct, sobriety and strict obedience to Nightingale.[9] Expectations such as these would continue as nursing developed into the twentieth century. But more importantly, they would provide the basis for the nursing that emerged in Canada.

Nightingale's legacy also extended into the area of the functions of the nurse, particularly in terms of the differentiation between nursing tasks and those tasks assigned to the physician. In her 1859 publication, <u>Notes on Nursing: What it is and What it is Not</u>, she clearly delineated the boundary between medicine and nursing. Nurses were to observe the patient and then to report those findings to the physician. She cautioned her readers against the "danger of physicking" and emphasized that "nursing ... is to put the patient in the best condition for nature to act upon him."[10] In spite of these efforts, territorial tension between medicine and nursing did develop. Nightingale was often moved to justify nursing education in the face of threatened opposition from the medical profession. Her cautious approach began in Scutari when a flood of sick suddenly burst into the Crimean hospital. When the means of the hospital were not able to meet the need, the physicians turned to Nightingale. Up to that point, Nightingale and her nurses had waited patiently for permission from the military physicians to care for the soldiers. This was the foundation on which she based her view of nursing and in August 1867, she noted that:

> we will never undertake the training of women as either physicians or surgeons. What we aim at is simply making them disciplined intelligent useful nurses ... to improve hospital nursing.[11]

In short, the role of the nurse was to be subordinate to the medical profession.

One last element of Nightingale's legacy for nursing was the religious fervour with which she infused the vocation. She viewed nursing as the performance of God's work. Such "work" could only be done by modest, temperate women who were daughters of God. Prayer was fundamental to the maintenance of this unblemished character and singing instructions were included in the training of Nightingale's nurses in order to stop "any temptation to bad language."[12] The important role religion held in Nightingale's view of nursing is strongly exemplified in her reflections following the unexpected death of Agnes Elizabeth Jones, one of Nightingale's star pupils:

> In less than three years – the time generally given to the ministry on earth of that Saviour whom she so earnestly strove closely to follow – she did all this. She had the gracefulness, the wit, the unfailing cheerfulness – qualities so remarkable but so much overlooked in our Saviour's life. She had the absence of all asceticism, or "mortification," for mortification's sake, which characterized His work, and any real work in the present day as in His day.[13]

Nightingale accompanied religious fervour with a morality that elevated the occupation to the level of a spiritual calling rather than that of a simple vocation. Nightingale admonished a group of her St. Thomas probationers that nursing, as a special call, needs a religious basis because the practice of nursing has a moral influence.[14] The nurse's "moral influence" would be exerted on those individuals situated in the hospital ward, thereby, transferring work previously done by the church into a hospital ward setting. As Nightingale asserted:

> Will He say to us some day; Well done, thou good and faithful Nurse; my ward was kept clean, and wholesome, and in order and quiet; my patients done by, as thou wouldst have done it for me; and a good example was set to all around; and Nurses are being trained up for me in my Probationers?[15]

Indeed, for Nightingale, the hospital ward was "God's kingdom on earth."

This close affiliation between the work of nursing and God's ministry brought acceptability to nursing. Consequently, Nightingale set the stage for nursing to be viewed as a spiritual vocation for suitable young women who would be trained, if they were not already, to be proper young ladies. Further, these nurses were expected to be obedient, loyal, dutiful, sober, moral, and to ground their practice of nursing in their deep religious faith. The Nightingale perspective was no doubt a reaction to the mid-nineteenth century negative image of nursing. What it succeeded in doing was sanction nursing as an appropriate career that enabled Victorian women to enter the working world. Nightingale also provided a respectable foundation on which nursing would build.

As nursing grew in respectability, hospitals became more acceptable to society as well. And as the domain of medical science, they were the institutions to look to for the treatment of illness and disease. By 1893, the popularity of hospitals had grown considerably. Isabel Hampton, an American nursing leader, observed that:

All classes of the population were entering hospitals ... not "paupers" only as in quite recent times; that hospitals must be responsible for disease prevention and health teaching, as well as for sick care; that they must collaborate much more closely with health departments in the protection of the public health and with educational institutions in the teaching of physicians and nurses.[16]

Hospitals thus became the environment in which nurses were trained. Nightingale believed that there should be:

a common nursing home in the hospital for hospital nurses and for probationer nurses; a common home for private nurses during intervals of engagements ... [that] under loving, trained, moral, and religious, as well as technical superintendence, ... [so] as to keep the tone of the inmates with constant supply of all material wants and constant sympathy.[17]

Therefore, living space was allocated in the teaching hospitals for the use of student nurses. In this environment, nurses were socialized to fulfill the Nightingale 'lady nurse' image.

The reforming temperament of the times reinforced this change and in turn this contributed to a change in the attitude towards women. Many young women had become frustrated with the limitations that the earlier societal convention had placed on them. Therefore, a significant labour pool was now available. The Nightingale educational model for nurses offered these women an opportunity to expand their horizons without threatening the current view of women. The fact that Nightingale's chief principle was "the entire subordination of the nursing corps to the medical staff" assured everyone that those women who ventured into nursing would always 'know their place'.[18] This further suggests that as long as nursing activities were subordinate to that of the physician and conducted under his supervision, the work was acceptable. This cautious beginning adhered satisfactorily to contemporary standards society held for late-nineteenth century women.

Initially, Nightingale's ideas were brought to Canada by Nightingale graduates who were employed in Montreal and Hamilton to establish schools of nursing. Hospitals promoted the notion that "a good nurse must be a good woman" in order to attract respectable women to the profession. Due to the risks encountered in a hospital setting, it was believed that there was no doubt that women in hospital life required more assistance to maintain their morality than women in family life or in domestic service.[19] Therefore the discipline administered in the nurses' home was a key element in the battle against immorality.

Dr. Theophilus Mack founded the first training school for nurses in Canada at the St. Catharine's General Hospital, in 1873. He imported six or eight nurses who had worked with Nightingale to establish the school under the motto "Where there is no woman a sick man groans."[20] The hospital administration expected each student to adhere to the rules and regulations of the school thus binding her to a three-year contract. The following excerpts from the school's prospectus reflect the Nightingale influence regarding the need for Christian charity, obedience, and conformity in all nursing students:

> ... Every woman entering the service must give satisfactory evidence of good character and Christian conduct, and of having received the elements of a plain English education. ... An implicit submission to the discipline of the Home and Hospital and obedience to those in authority there, as well as a strict conformity to rules and regulations, will be exacted.[21]

This school was the first successful school in Canada modeled on Nightingale's school in St. Thomas' hospital in London.

The Montreal General Hospital School of Nursing, established around the same time, did not meet with similar success. Up to this point, the Montreal General Hospital had not considered nursing to be of any significance. But, in 1875, this same hospital enticed Miss Mary Machin, a Nightingale-trained nurse, to Montreal. The hospital administrators promised her a new hospital and sought her advice regarding the proposed building plans. Machin left for Montreal in August 1875 and after settling in, reported to Nightingale that the situation was "tolerable."

This "tolerable" situation soon became "treacherous" following the completion of a report inquiring into "increased expenditures with a view to retrenching." The report concluded that Machin was the cause of the extravagance and that any outlay not accounted for was laid to her charge. Furthermore, Machin reported back to Nightingale, since the Lady Superintendent was:

a superfluous expence[sic] & that as the Training School was their principal object in bringing me out & it had been found impracticable (this fact also news to me) therefore it would not be desirable to renew any engagement with Miss Machin.[22]

Machin had considerable support in the hospital from both the administration and the medical people, as well as the citizenry of Montreal. Indeed, everyone was determined to treat her judiciously and with fairness because of the improvements she had made to the hospital. The ensuing investigations and debate led to enormous public pressure in support of Miss Machin but she was left feeling unnerved.[23] Ultimately, she was exonerated.

In spite of her apparent victory, Machin was not comfortable remaining in Montreal and decided to submit her resignation in June, 1878. On hearing this, her staff followed her lead and declined the Committee's invitation to stay.[24]

In spite of this shaky beginning, hospitals, both large and small, emerged across Canada between 1890 and 1910 and, as in the case of Victoria's Royal Jubilee Hospital, many of the directors decided to establish a school for training nurses in connection with the institution. In order to attract candidates, newspaper accounts described nursing glowingly as a notable occupation that brought into play the highest and best powers an individual can possess. The avocation of the nurse was depicted as an act of moral heroism. Hospital managers touted nursing as a "noble profession" to entice students to their schools but gave these women a vocational preparation. These apprenticeship-training programs were simply a solution to the financial problems that the hospitals were experiencing at the time. Indeed, by 1909, seventy training schools in Canada were attached to hospitals.[25]

Any fears society might have had regarding the presence of young ladies in the hospital environment were alleviated by the respectability that now surrounded nursing service. Parents could be assured of the fact that the work of nursing was absolutely necessary for the continued health of the patient and that the propriety of those young nurses would be maintained within the residential setting. Although opportunities in nursing offered nineteenth-century women an occupation outside of the home environment, the nursing education that emerged was simply exploitation of their work.

As the need for nursing services escalated, the demand for trained nurses exceeded the supply, therefore nursing schools across Canada multiplied because it was necessary for each hospital to recruit and train its own nursing staff. The training school for nurses was established to provide nursing service in the hospital, give the medical profession intelligent and skilful cooperation, and offer instruction in the art of nursing to women who were fitted by nature and education. Therefore, it was important to promote nursing in such a way that it would appeal to acceptable candidates. A variety of publications elaborated on the type of woman most suited to perform the functions of a nurse. That woman was:

> A young woman of intelligent face, neat apparel, and quiet demeanor ... Her skillful[sic] hand prepared the food, her watchful eye anticipated every want. She was calm, patient, and sympathizing; ... She did not stoop to simulate an affection she did not feel, nor to express hopes of recovery that could not be realized ... She met emergency with knowledge and unruffled spirit. To the physician she proved an invaluable assistant, executing his orders intelligently, and recording accurately the various symptoms as they developed. She watched the temperature of the room as closely as that of the patient.[26]

This suggests that the 'ideal nurse' was to be a paragon of virtue who was loyal and self-sacrificing. Along with the required altruism, intelligence, skill, and hard work, the reward for performing backbreaking, hard, earnest work was the "sweet smile" of a convalescing patient. The Canadian Nurse encouraged and supported these notions in an article that noted:

> Above all we are women of character. Loyal pure in thought and life, patient, kind, and sympathetic, not lacking in forbearance, controlling ourselves in the most trying circumstances, bright, cheerful and entertaining while at the same time serious and firm when necessary, not forgetting that tact is one of the essentials in the makeup of the nurse. Lastly: Our compensation apart from a financial one, is the consciousness of duty well performed, as well as the heartfelt gratitude of our patient and our patient's friends.[27]

Success of this promotional scheme was obvious in that nursing attracted more and more respectable women.

The medical profession reinforced these ideas as well. Since in the early days of nursing training, there were few, if any, nurses who had the requisite knowledge to teach students,

◖dividual members of the medical profession took on the task of ◖ecturing students. In their lectures to student nurses, physicians frequently described those qualities that created a well-rounded, ideal nurse. In a series of four lectures presented to the student nurses at St. Michael's Hospital in Toronto, the physician used his first lecture to address the question of "The Nurse Herself." The remaining three lectures discussed the patient, various operations, and nursing duties in the Operating Room. Throughout the lecture on "The Nurse Herself," the physician-teacher insisted that his "ideal nurse" be "essentially feminine, ... brave as a lion, and though duly vigilant, ha[ve] no fear of her own safety" and in the house of a poor man, shine like a ray of sunlight. He also cautioned his audience to remember "that a nurse is not a doctor and should never attempt to pass as one." Given the amount of information covered in this publication, the ten pages that were taken up with "The Nurse Herself" would suggest that for nursing generally, the personality characteristics of the potential candidates were of the utmost importance. According to the medical profession, "the true nurse is born, not made. [S]ympathy is more the property of women than men and so it is that women always make the best nurses."[28]

In order to attract young women to the hospitals, romanticized notions accompanied the promotional rhetoric of physicians. Physicians painted themselves as powerless without the valuable assistance of nurses. This view contained elements of self-interest because as hospitals multiplied, the patient-load increased, and Canadian physicians looked to nurses, trained in the Nightingale system, to meet the increased demands. In this way the Nightingale legacy continued in Canada, and the medical profession would remain forever obligated to Florence Nightingale and her system of training nurses.

Socialization of the student nurse was a key element of the Nightingale nursing education system. Upon completion of the hospital program, the graduate was admonished to carry on the well-established Nightingale nursing tradition. One of the first graduates from the Montreal General Hospital remembered the Superintendent of Nurses' parting words to her class:

> Young ladies, you are the pioneers in the field of professional nursing. It will be your task to educate the public and to blaze the trail for those who will follow you. Many of the untrained nurses have been eating with the maids. Make arrangements when you enter a home to have your meals served on a tray. Be dignified and wise ...[29]

Therefore, the training of young women for nursing was also a socialization process that produced young ladies who showed wifely obedience to the physician, motherly devotion to the patient, and a firm mistress-servant discipline to those below her on the hospital or home bureaucratic ladder.

By 1910, the Nightingale legacy for nursing had been well entrenched in Canada. Adherence to her principles was reflected in nursing education, desirable attributes for the nurse, and the socialization process. Furthermore, nursing leaders incorporated these traditions in the hierarchical, organizational structures they created.

Indeed, the developments in Canadian nursing during this time period were ushered in by a group of women who conformed to the social purity collective described by historian Mariana Valverde. Nursing leaders of the day shared very specific class, gender, and ethnic characteristics and generally supported the domination of Anglo-Saxon middle class males. These males allowed women of the right class and ethnicity a substantial role in society, as long as they were dependent on male protection.[30] Nursing's birth and early development did occur under the protective eye of the medical profession and the hospital administrators. The leaders came from families of "the right class and ethnicity," and held similar cultural values to that of the dominant group. This was clearly true for M.A. Snively and G.E. Livingstone, two early leaders in nursing education. Snively's parents were of Swiss and Irish protestant descent and

Livingston's parents were English and protestant.[31] This would be in keeping, therefore, with the white Anglo-Saxon and Protestant background of the dominant male group.

At the same time, this mutually agreeable situation allowed these nursing leaders the freedom to direct the development of the nursing vocation with little or no significant interference. Since both nurses and physicians agreed on the ultimate goal, their activities interacted and complemented each other. As long as the goal was the social purification of Canadians, any "regulation" that was incorporated was used to preserve and shape, not suppress or dominate.[32] Therefore, participation in these activities allowed nursing to gain acceptance and legitimacy.

Mary Agnes Snively personified the social purity collective. Once described as the "Mother of Nurses" in Canada, she identified three requisites for success in nursing as "self-sacrifice, loyalty to duty, and heroism."[33] As a result of her efforts, the Canadian National Association of Trained Nurses was formed in 1908. Under her leadership (1908-1912), the Canadian National Association of Trained Nurses (CNATN) supported Snively's motto, "Into the Future Open a Better Way."[34] A motto such as this mirrored the optimistic view of the future generally held by all Canadians.

Snively's successful introduction of Canadian nursing to the International Council of Nurses in 1909 indicates the apparent desire of nurses to come together on an international level. At each meeting, Ethel Bedford-Fenwick, British founder of the International Council of Nurses, presented a watchword that was to guide the direction nursing took during the intervening years before the next meeting. The three words for the first decade of the twentieth century were "work," "courage," and "life."[35] All three words suggest a need to inspire and motivate members of the vocation to a 'noble calling', which now emerged as a new profession for women.

It was later noted by the editor of a historical publication celebrating the fiftieth anniversary of the nursing school established at the Toronto General Hospital that:

> The main development in the general history of nursing during the first ten years of the twentieth century was the employment of special nurses in hospitals. This was another indication of the changed attitude of the public towards the business of nursing the sick, recognizing it as skilled work, and demanding the thoroughly trained expert in cases where special care was needed ... The field of nursing was won; and the drive to establish it, and settle it in its place in the life of the community was over. What remained was to experiment with its functioning, both inside the hospital and out.[36]

These developments would not have occurred without the support of Canadian society.

By 1910, the groundwork had been laid for the future growth of nursing in Canada. This occurred in a climate of change, reform, and a growing faith in medical science. As Canadians turned to medicine for solutions, the medical profession shifted its practice from the office in the community to the larger setting of the hospital. The mid-nineteenth century hospital and associated staff had a reputation that would not attract anyone outside of the indigent to it therefore, improvements had to be made. New hospitals were constructed and staffed by nurses who conformed to the Nightingale 'lady-nurse'. The conformity, or socialization process, occurred within the Nightingale nursing education system that was imported to Canadian nursing schools by Nightingale nurses. In order to make nursing attractive and acceptable to the parents of potential candidates, the vocation was painted in terms that would appeal to the values of a late-Victorian society. Although productive in terms of recruitment, the ideal characteristics of nursing that were promoted resulted in the emergence of a spiritual vocation that was subservient to the medical profession and dependent on the good will of the larger society. At the same time, Canadian nursing leaders displayed vision and political astuteness in their strategies. They not only succeeded in attracting large numbers of young women to nursing but assured themselves of increasing their power as a group that would be in a position to direct their future through their national and organizational efforts.

CHAPTER ONE NOTES

[1] Charles P.Cleaves, "The Nurse," CN, Vol.I, No.1, March, 1905, p. 73.

[2] Ramsay Cook, Regenerators, p. 6.

[3] Health and Home, February, 1884. p. 12.

[4] _____, "An Account of the origin, Rise and Progress of the Montreal General Hospital," Reprinted from The Literary Repository, No.XX, Vol.IV, February,1825, p. 16.

[5] Quoted in Janice Acton et al., Women at Work: Ontario 1850-1930, (Toronto: Canadian Women's Educational Press, 1974), p. 136.

[6] Quoted in Janice Acton et al., Women at Work, p. 131.

[7] Sir James Alexander Grant, "Address Delivered before the Canadian Medical Association," August 6,1873, Saint John, New Brunswick, p.8, CIHM #06520.

[8] Lytton Strachey, Eminent Victorians, (New York: Putnam, 1918), p. 125.

[9] Florence Nightingale, "Memorandum of Agreement," in "Correspondence of Sir John Hall," British Library (BL), London, England, MSS 39867, FF105.

[10] Florence Nightingale, Notes on Nursing: What it is and What it is Not, (Philadelphia: Lippincott, 1859), pp. 131-136.

[11] Nightingale Papers, Nightingale to Recipient, August,1867, BL, London, MSS47767, 15-16.

[12] "Nightingale letter to the Edinburgh Infirmary Nurses," December 6, 1873, Canadian Nurses Association Archives (CNAA), Ottawa. Florence Nightingale, "Suggestions for the Improvement of the Nursing Service of Hospitals and on the Method of Training Nurses for the Sick Poor" in Report on Cubic Space in Metropolitan Workhouses, 1867, p. 5.

[13] Florence Nightingale, "Una," Good Words, June, 1868.

[14] Sir Edward Cook, The Life of Florence Nightingale, Vol.II. (New York: The MacMillan Company, 1942), p. 263.

[15] F. Nightingale, "Letter to the Nurses of the Edinburgh Infirmary," (Edinburgh, Scotland, 1873), p. 2.

[16] Isabel Hampton et al., Nursing of the Sick, Imternational Congress of Charities, Correction and Philanthropy, 1893, p. xviii.

[17] Ibid., p. 32.

[18] Franklin H. North, "A New Profession for Women," Century Illustrated Monthly Magazine, Vol.XXV, November 1882, p. 39.

[19] Nightingale Papers, 1874, BL, ADD 47767, FF.28.

[20] The Mack Training School for Nurses, St Catharine's General Hospital, 1874-1934. p. 6, CNAA.

[21] "First Annual Report, July 1st, 1875, The St. Catharines Training School and Nurses' Home in connection with the General and Marine Hospital," p. 20, CNAA.

[22] Nightingale Papers, Nightingale-Machin Correspondence, June 26, 1875, BL, ADD 47745, FF. 55-58, September 19, 1877, BL, FF.92. August, 1875, FF.49-50, October 16, 1875, FF.63-65. FF.93.

[23] Ibid., October 19,,1877, BL, FF.96-101.Ibid., November 5, 1877, BL, FF.102-104.

[24] Ibid., June 6, 1878, BL, FF.108-111.

[25] Anne Pearson, The Royal Jubilee Hospital School of Nursing 1891-1982, (Victoria: The Alumnae Association of the Royal Jubilee School of Nursing, 1985), p. 1.

[26] Pauline O. Jardine, "An Urban Middle-Class Calling: Women and the Emergence of Modern Nursing Education at Toronto General Hospital 1881-1914," Urban History Review, Vol. XVII, No.3 (February, 1989), p. 179, p. 38.

[27] Janet G.McNeill, "On Nurses and Nursing," CN, Vol. VI, No.1, January 1910, p. 110.

[28] James F.W.Ross, Four lectures Delivered to the Nurses of St. Michael's Hospital Toronto, (Toronto: William Briggs, 1901), p. 13-14, 5, 9. University of Toronto Archives (UTA), Toronto, B85-0022/001.

[29] Quoted in Acton et al., p. 139.

[30] Mariana Valverde, The Age of Light, Soap and Water, (Toronto: McClelland & Stewart Inc., 1991), p. 24, 33.

[31] Jean E. Browne, "Daughter of Canada," CN, Vol.XX, No.10, October 1924, p.618 and E. Francis Upton, "Miss Livingston," CN, Vol.XXI, No.6, June 1925, p.295. Snively founded the Toronto General Hospital Training School for nurses and Livingstone established one at the Montreal General Hospital.

[32] Valverde, p. 33.

[33] _____, A Brief History of the Canadian Nurses Association, (Ottawa: Canadian Nurses Association, ND), p. 19, and Jean E. Browne, "In

Memoriam: Mary Agnes Snively," CN, Vol. XXIX, No.11, November 1933, pp. 567-570.

[34] Dorothy Meilicke, "CNA Presidents, 1908-1980: Beginning Biographies and Presidential Themes," unpublished notes, February, 1981, CNAA, Ottawa.

[35] Daisy Caroline Bridges, A History of the International Council of Nurses 1899-1964, (Toronto: J.B.Lippincott Company, 1967), pp. 17-21,25,31.

[36] Margaret Isabel Lawrence, ed., History: The School for Nurses, Toronto General Hospital, (Toronto: Toronto General Hospital, ND), p. 23.

Chapter Two

WAR AND EPIDEMIC: 1914-1919

During the years 1914 to 1919, Canadian nursing continued its transformation from spiritual vocation to secular profession. This transformation corresponded with a growing self-confidence in nursing that grew out of the increasing value the public placed on nursing service. World War I and the Spanish Flu Epidemic had resulted in an escalating need for nursing expertise, a need that nurses filled. In meeting this need, nurses created a situation in which the activities of the nurse and those of Canadians became intensely involved. Nursing, therefore, continued to evolve as a reflection of, and a response to, those concerns of the larger society within which it existed.

The willingness with which nurses responded to the war and the flu contributed to their growing importance in the health care scheme. During World War I, nurses committed themselves to caring for Canadians both at home and overseas. More than 2,000 nurses enlisted in 1914 and at the close of the war, 52 had been killed. Similarly, during the flu epidemic, nurses participated fully in the care of the sick and trained volunteer help to meet the desperate need for nursing services. The heightened profile that nurses gained brought nursing out from behind the walls of the hospital and nurses' home and placed it firmly in the public eye.

Furthermore, nurses and the nursing leaders were united in their undertaking to assist Canadians during these two crises and

Canadians rewarded their efforts by further enlisting their assistance in matters related to health. This goal was aided by the broadening conception of the nurse's role in health promotion and disease prevention that was added to her function of caring for the sick. Hospitals and training schools had already become accepted in the community but public health now emerged as a critical issue. Indeed, it was reported to the New Brunswick branch of the Canadian Red Cross that participants at the Conference of the Great Powers at Cannes heard that:

> The loss of human life through war, and the much greater loss through the epidemic of influenza in 1918 (it was estimated that 20,000,000 lives were lost in that epidemic), as well as the appalling degree of physical unfitness revealed by medical examinations of recruits for the services, constituted by far the most important problem for discussion. It was decided that there should be a great world-wide public health organization to help bring up the standards of physical and mental fitness of the world.[1]

Consequently, the public health movement, in which nursing came to be a fundamentally important component, grew in significance.

All of these events contributed in large measure to a growing self-confidence among nurses themselves, which, in turn, sparked the beginnings of assertiveness. During these years, nursing leaders addressed such issues as provincial registration for nurses, nursing education, municipal funding for hospitals, affiliation with the Canadian National Council of Women, and the eight-hour day for nurses. Therefore, all four criteria for professionalism as outlined at the outset of this study are identifiable. In fact, 1919 ushered in the first university nursing education program and this represented a major step towards professionalism. Finally, throughout this eventful period, nursing met little opposition from the medical profession; indeed, that voice was quiet.

Immediately prior to the outbreak of the First World War, nursing leaders expressed concern regarding the gradually declining numbers of eligible candidates entering nursing and the deteriorating standard of care offered by the nurses. They identified several trends that would eventually strain the ability of the existing system to cope with the needs of the public. Such trends included "the widening horizons of medical practice, growing public consciousness of the need to extend and improve the care provided by the state for its citizens, and public recognition of the need for improvement in all educational systems."[2] Therefore, the Canadian Association of Trained Nurses created a Special Committee to investigate nursing education. The Committee included representatives from the University of Toronto and the University of Manitoba. In 1914, they submitted their report. The main recommendation was to "establish nurse training schools or colleges in connection with the educational system of each province." This would suggest limited support for improvements in nursing education but the final recommendation offered a clear indication of just how limited that support was. The report advised "that the whole matter be considered calmly - not from the personal standpoint, but from that of 'Summum Bonum'."[3] In 1914, however, the 'Summum Bonum' or "highest good" with which the community was concerned was the threat of war with Germany, not nursing education.

The outbreak of World War I took the attention of the nursing elite away from the question of education to focus on more practical concerns. In fact, Gibbon and Mathewson observe that within 3 weeks after the declaration of war, thousands of nurses volunteered for service overseas.[4] Canadian nurses had already earned recognition for their military service. In 1904, nursing sisters were accorded the relative military rank of lieutenant thus making them the first group of women to be accorded a relative military rank.[5] Canadian nurses, along with Canadians in general, responded to the war effort to protect the British Empire against the German threat.

Indeed in 1917, the Canadian National Association of Trained Nurses passed a resolution offering the services of Canadian nurses :

> to be utilized in such a manner as the federal government shall deem best in the present national crisis ... If ... conscription of nurses should appear necessary or desirable, we stand prepared to answer the call.[6]

They clearly lived up to their reputation. As Agnes J. Macleod, Director of Nursing Service in the Department of Veteran's Affairs, later recalled in <u>The Canadian Nurse</u>:

> Canadian Nursing Sisters were exposed to all the rigors of war and several lost their lives in the bombing of Canadian hospitals. The experiences of the sisters with the Mediterranean Expeditionary Force were very harrowing. The heat, the rain, the pests and resultant infections were hard to bear.[7]

The war not only brought changes to the political role of women but also "accelerated trends that had been observed in prewar Canada," such as an increase in the percentage of women in professional areas. Historians have noted that "these professional jobs were mainly in the fields of teaching and nursing" and that "they did give women a mobility, economic and geographical, which they had lacked in the nineteenth century."[8] The War offered nursing a breadth of opportunity heretofore unimagined. These wartime experiences presented nurses with numerous opportunities to work, often without medical supervision, away from home in situations where their efforts were not only important but validated as such, daily.

One such nurse, Anne E. Ross, outlined her experience in a sixteen-page diary that gives an accurate depiction of what most nurses confronted after joining the Canadian Expeditionary Forces. Anne Ross joined the military in March 1915 and returned to Canada following Armistice, in 1918. Her direct

Fortify Your System
Against the "Flu"

In these days of the "Flu" epidemic every man, woman and child should take immediate precautions to safeguard their health.

Medical authorities agree that the only sure defence against the attacks of "Flu" germs is—to keep your system in sound condition at all times. To do this a body building tonic is essential—and in

O'Keefe's

IMPERIAL BEVERAGES
Ale, Lager and Stout

you will find the tonic necessary.

O'Keefe's beverage tonics contain the nutriment and strength giving properties of well-brewed malt and hops. Nothing harmful is contained in any O'Keefe brew. The invigorating tonic benefits result from the nutritious food values contained in the beverages.

Order O'Keefe's today and fortify your system against the "Flu."

Ask for O'Keefe's at Restaurants, Cafes, Inns, Hotels, etc., or order direct from your grocer.

O'Keefe Brewery Co., Limited
TORONTO, ONT.   Main 4202.

Canada Food Board License 1-15-101

Newspaper advertisement reflecting the 'need for a cure' during the
Spanish Influenza Epidemic following WWI.

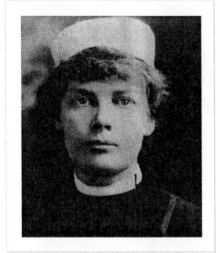

LEFT: Ethel Johns, Director of the School of Nursing at the University of British Columbia during the establishment of the Baccalaureate degree 'sandwich' program. (Courtesy Helen K. Mussallem Library)

BOTTOM: Public health clinic during the 'roaring twenties' in Calgary. (Courtesy Calgary General Hospital Alumnae)

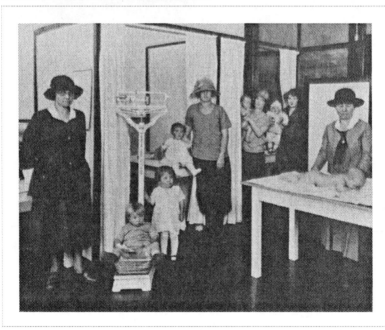

narrative lacks melodrama but is informative. Although most nurses offered their services willingly, they approached their departure overseas with trepidation. The following anecdote reflects the danger that accompanied sailing across the Atlantic:

> We were put on board the SS Hesperian about 4PM and had dinner. Our ship sailed Sunday May 2nd at 6AM. May 10th we arrived safely in Liverpool. The Lousitania sailed from New York after we did and had been sunk in the North Sea. Our course was slightly changed and Capt. Main had remained in the chart room the last 36 hours of our trip on the look for submarines. The Hesperian made one more trip across and was sunk by submarines.[9]

This anecdote is brief and direct and reflects the pragmatic, unsentimental attitude this particular nurse adopted as she embarked on her overseas experience. This attitude was shared by many of the nursing sisters in spite of the continuous danger they faced.[10]

Anne Ross's nursing service took her from England to the Aegean on hospital ships, and to Europe where she provided nursing care in stationary hospitals close to the Front. Throughout these travels, she would have experienced fatigue and exposure to various infectious diseases; therefore, it is not surprising to read that she was unable to resist amoebic dysentery. Following her recuperation in England, she returned to duty at Taplow, an experience that she described as her happiest days overseas.

During the winter of 1916/17, however, Ross was sent to France and the hardships associated with the front. For her, "life again was different" which was her rather understated description of life at the Front. At times she sounds almost bored with the monotony of the annual drives made by the German army as she notes:

Time went on. 1917 passed[,] our work was closer to the front than at Taplow. we would evacuate, receive a convoy and so carried on for another year. March always meant a big drive. Xmas again and ... we come to the big drive in March 1918. The Germans were pushing on to Paris and Amiens.[11]

Similarly, zeppelin attacks and gas attacks were commonplace and dealt with in a professionally appropriate manner. Ross had obviously adjusted to her wartime duties in the three years since her departure from Canada and this competency would bring her additional respect on her return home.

Anne Ross referred specifically to her nursing duties only once and this was following her appointment as Night Supervisor in August, 1918:

The duties of Night Supervisor are many and responsibilities heavy. Night always brought dread of hemorrhages. 4AM being the zero hour and most hemorrhages occured[sic] at that time. I had to call Orderly Officer, Padre in case of death, Operating Room staff and meet all emergencies. 36 wards - 40pts. in each ward, overflow in tents up to 700 in avg.[12]

This was an incredible responsibility for a single nurse. Anne E. Ross appeared to cope very well. Much of her work would have been accomplished without the direct supervision of a physician and would contribute to the production of a strong independent nurse. This strength of character was also clear in her description of her return to Canada in 1919: "Called to London and assigned to boat to sail next day. Sailing cancelled [sic] - strike - sailed in May - arrived in Quebec June 3rd - Home June 5th - Back on duty June 29th in Kingston."[13]

The fact that she returned to work only twenty-four days after arriving home from a four-year stint overseas is quite remarkable. This is the profile of a nurse who had developed a considerable amount of self-confidence and strength from her wartime experience and was able to meet any and all tasks that she faced.

In addition to gaining self-confidence, nurses returning from their overseas experience became a close-knit, strongly unified group with a continuing respect for sacrifice. Hierarchy as is demonstrated in Anne Ross's description of her Matron's dying moments did not limit this unity:

> Our dearly beloved matron ... I spoke of at the beginning. Our matron Mrs. Jaggard Canadian born and trained as a nurse, wife of a President of one of the W.S. Railways gave up a life of luxury to serve her motherland. It was my privilege to nurse her in her dying hours - In her we lost a friend. One who was well able to give us good advice.[14]

This anecdote reflects a commitment to the war effort but it also exemplifies the camaraderie and loyalty nurses held for each other. Matron-in-Chief MacDonald noted that none of the nursing sisters complained or asked for transfers to less dangerous areas. In fact "it was well recognized throughout the Canadian Army Medical Corps that the ambition of its Nursing Sisters was to carry on their work regardless of personal danger, and as close to the firing as permitted."[15] The desperate situations encountered in this particular war and the public acclamation of the heroic efforts of the nurses elevated the reputation of nursing in general and contributed to unity and solidarity within Canadian nursing.

Moreover, the reputation of Canadian nurses was such that they were called upon to assist in the nursing of His Majesty King George V, whose horse had reared and fallen upon him while reviewing Canadian troops. Two Canadian nurses returned to Buckingham Palace and continued to care for him during this "very long and tedious and painful illness" for which both nurses were awarded the Royal Victoria Order Silver Medal. As a result of their wartime efforts, Canadian nurses received a total of 905 decorations of one sort or another, proof of their growing serviceability to Canadians.[16] This enthusiastic response given the war effort by Canadian nurses promoted their cause further in the eyes of the Canadian public.

Although considerably less dramatic, nurses were active on the home front as well. The need for nurses overseas caused a marked depletion in personnel at home; therefore, students became the essential hospital staff, often with only a Lady Superintendent, a Day Supervisor, and a Night Supervisor to guide them. Sixteen-hour shifts were common with little, or no, time off. Many graduates were engaged in Private Duty work but, as in the case of the Calgary General Hospital, on their free days they turned up at the hospital to roll bandages and make dressings and received no pay for their services.[17] Nurses met and fulfilled all of the demands made of them during the war. Their success in this endeavour gave them considerable self-confidence. However, nobody expected another emergency to follow as quickly on the heels of the war as the flu epidemic did.

Once again, conditions called for nursing expertise. The relief that accompanied the ending of the war did not prepare Canadians for the influenza epidemic that returned home with the victorious Canadian Expeditionary Forces in 1918. Although initially viewed casually as some kind of infection, Spanish Flu quickly engendered fear throughout Canada with its rapid onset and death.

The "Spanish Flu" was as devastating in Canada as it was elsewhere. The Flu entered Canada on troop ships during the summer of 1918. Initially, the disease did not spread rapidly, however, it was obvious by the end of September that Canada had a problem. The epidemic adhered to historical tradition and traveled westerly across the country by means of the railway. This was a unique variety of flu in that it had a high morbidity rate and a much higher mortality rate than previously associated with flus. Moreover, "it also manifested the curious feature of killing, not the very young and the very old ... but healthy individuals in the prime of life."[18] By 1918, Spanish Influenza had affected one in every six Canadians and killed between thirty and fifty thousand people. Yet, in the majority of history books, it is not mentioned and in others, it is dismissed in a paragraph or two.[19] In spite of this dismissal, the flu constituted a major event in Canada, particularly for nursing.

The fear and panic that this tragedy generated spearheaded a campaign to recruit nurses as soon as possible. Lectures on nursing victims of the Spanish Flu were offered, for example, on the steps of the Ontario Legislature and reprinted in <u>The Toronto World</u> for "Young Lady Volunteers." This somewhat unusual approach was justified by the lecturer who cited the emergent nature of the situation. More importantly, it is clear that consensus existed regarding the need for nursing services. The physician who presented the lectures stated at the outset that:

> It is an absolute impossibility to make nurses or to give any complete idea of nursing in the course of three lectures, but I believe it is possible to give a sufficient description of certain essentials of the sick room, the preparation and care of the bed and of the general observation of the sick patient that will be of great benefit to anyone who has the time and will to help in this emergency.[20]

This opening statement was followed by basic but detailed instructions regarding "General Preparation for Nursing at Home." The importance of nursing care made rapid gains during this crisis. In Calgary, for example, the biggest single need at the time was for nurses. Special influenza hospitals were set up and "any nurse who could be spared went to help direct the nursing being done in the centres by teachers, housewives, and secretaries."[21]

Numerous advertisements appeared in newspapers across Canada with bold headlines such as, "Wanted, Volunteers!!" that were calling for volunteers to train and supply nursing assistance.[22] The Alberta Provincial Health Department provided similar information in the Calgary <u>Daily Herald</u> notice entitled, "Epidemic Influenza - Instructions Regarding care of Sick Persons," which offered information related to fresh air, rest, nourishment, and associated precautions.[23] In spite of this apparent reasoned approach, newspaper accounts fostered panic in headlines such as "Spanish Influenza Rages in Canada."[24] Quarantine, masks, and a variety of home-based remedies were recommended as protection against the deadly bug. The fear and desperation that existed among Canadians is further exemplified in one tragic news item entitled, "Took Wrong Crystals for Influenza." The item stated that:

> Dr. C.A. Jarvis, one of the best known optometrists in Canada, died instantly this morning through taking the wrong medicine for influenza. He was at his office and reached up for some crystals. Inadvertently he took those of cyanide potassium. Recognising his mistake he called to the staff to get a doctor, but expired almost immediately.[25]

This anecdote is a clear example of the panic that existed among Canadians at the time.

The flu epidemic did spur great activity among medical scientists and their institutions. Indeed, following the flu, significant steps were made in health care in Canada, particularly regarding the organization of health services. As noted by historian Janice Dickin-McGinnis:

> The International Red Cross gave the epidemic as one of three reasons for extending its activities into peacetime. In Canada, communities voted funds for hospitals that had somehow never seemed that urgent before. Calgary's civic elections at the beginning of December 1918 were dominated by health issues. Nova Scotia established a public health nursing course at Dalhousie University. And the United Farm Women's Association, meeting in Edmonton in January 1919, called for a system of medical and nursing aid

to provide adequate health care, especially in rural areas, and a federal department of health.[26]

Not surprisingly, the war and the flu focused more attention on the condition of public health and nurses participated in the discussion. The Victorian Order of Nurses wrote an article that directed the readers' attention to the urgent need in Canada for public health nurses. The writer noted that:

> We are informed by the Health authorities of the Western provinces, that there were more casualties from Influenza than from the war ... more babies die in Canada yearly, under one year old, from preventative causes, than soldiers have been killed any year during the war ... As an offset to this, the medical profession of all the social service organizations have begune[sic] to realize the great importance and necessity of the Public Health Nurse in combating these conditions.[27]

Together, the war and the flu not only brought nursing service to the attention of everyone but also pointed to two areas in which Canadian society was deficient. One was the poor level of physical health of Canadians and the other related to the poor health of the community. The former showed up among the Canadian Expeditionary Forces and the latter was emphasized in the spread of the flu. Both of these issues were manifestations of pre-war socio-economic dislocations and the post-war statistical revelation that "half of the adult males of military age were physically unfit." This situation was exacerbated by a gradual build-up of industrial unrest as thousands of returning soldiers poured into the country seeking work or health treatment. The arrival of new immigrants searching for a new life along with the materialization of a multitude of war widows, contributed further to the creation of additional social dislocations.[28]

A public health movement had existed for some time but according to historian Neil Sutherland, it was most effective in the lives of children.[29] As such, one particular location that attracted the reformers attention was that of the school. The goal was to improve the health of the school children and to reduce mortality among infants and young children. Reformers were convinced that the nurse played a significant role in this venture and by 1914, the Toronto School Health Department, for example, employed a total of thirty-seven full-time school nurses.[30] The nurse became a health educator and instructed Canadian women regarding the maintenance of a healthy home environment. These activities expanded to create a system that made the nurse "not only a skilled agency for the relief of suffering, but a teacher of sanitary and healthful living, and a power for the prevention of disease."[31] Thus nursing became 'an interpretive link between scientific advances and society in the public health movement.

The Canadian National Association for Trained Nurses accepted this role and in 1914, formed a "standing committee on public health nursing and social service" that was to have provincial representation and report regularly to the national executive.[32] Articles appeared in The Canadian Nurse that gave further evidence of a mediatory image:

> This [public health campaign] she [public health nurse] undertakes through propaganda of education. Whereas science has pointed out many causes and many remedies, science alone ... is of little or no value to the masses of our people ... We must look for an interpreter of science. This is the most important role perhaps that the public health is to play ... She is an interpreter of science to her people. More than that she is an interpreter of her people and their needs to law makers and to others of political influence.[33]

In 1917, the national association supported this gradually expanding role of the nurse in public health reform by adopting the recommendation that public health nursing include:

> Tuberculosis and industrial nursing; sanitary inspection, when carried on by nurses; pre-natal and child welfare

nursing; school nursing; hospital social service; or any other form of social work for which a nurse's training is essential.[34]

Clearly, the extension of nursing into these areas placed nurses in the mainstream of society and reflected the professional aspirations held by the nursing leaders.

Nursing was no longer restricted to the care of the sick but was developing further into the guardianship of public health. This shift to prevention was closely connected to the rapid growth in scientific knowledge that pointed to "the importance of the conquest of disease by preventive medicine and surgery."[35] Society, nursing and medicine all agreed so that the next step was left to the politicians.

The federal government addressed the situation in 1919 and established a Department of Health to administer all matters and questions relating to the promotion or preservation of the health and social welfare of Canadians. At the same time, a Dominion Council of Health was created whose task it was to develop health policies, among other things. An expert, or scientific adviser in the field of public health was also appointed. Public health units staffed by a physician with public health training, a sanitary inspector, and one or more public health nurses emerged across Canada. Indeed, British Columbia claims to have been the first province to organize a Health Centre with a Public Health Nursing Service in 1919, in Saanich.[36] Furthermore, in 1919, the Canadian National Association for Trained Nurses concluded that "the need that exists in every locality in Canada is the need for nurses qualified for leadership in the public health field, and for women to supplement nursing care in the homes."[37]

In 1919, the Canadian Red Cross joined forces with those looking for increased numbers of public health nurses. It would appear that the influenza epidemic motivated the search. The Red Cross offered scholarship funding for diploma courses in public health nursing to the universities of Toronto, McGill, British Columbia, Alberta, and Dalhousie. The Red Cross specified the qualifications for successful applicants and stated that one-half of these scholarships would be granted to Canadian nurses who had served overseas, provided there was a sufficient number of satisfactory applicants from the group.[38] This vote of confidence offered by the Red Cross Society points to the ascent of nursing both in the eyes of the public and in those of a related professional organization which would then nourish a developing assertiveness in Canadian nursing.

Nurses across Canada had been quietly but tenaciously, working towards registration legislation for the profession. By 1918, the nursing profession in Canada had successfully obtained Registration legislation in five provinces: Nova Scotia, Manitoba, New Brunswick, Alberta, and British Columbia. These Registration Acts were the means by which nurses took control of admission standards for training and the length of the training. In Alberta, a 1919 amendment was passed to the Registration Act "placing the nurses association among other professional associations under the control of the University of Alberta." This new status brought standardization to nursing education in Alberta, in that it was necessary henceforth, that a nurse write qualifying examinations set by the University in order to earn the right to use the initials 'RN' after her name.[39]

Ontario nurses had been moving in this direction, but to date, were unsuccessful. Indeed, a letter appeared in The Globe that described nursing as "the most autocratic and highly paid body of women in Canada."[40] The letter-writer decried the fact that there was no disciplinary arm in the Ontario nursing profession. A spokesperson for the Canadian National Association of Trained Nurses responded to the newspaper that:

> Blame must be laid at the door of those who have persistently refused State Educational and Legal recognition of the nursing profession in Ontario. In some of the other provinces Provincial Registration of Nurses exists and in the

event of misconduct, the license of the offender can be revoked and her name struck from the list.[41]

In spite of this support, Ontario nurses were not successful in their pursuit until 1922.

Provincially and nationally, Canadian nursing leaders were unanimous in their support of professional registration. This unity had grown out of the national organization's observation that "with unity among nurses, and a thorough understanding on their part of all that registration involves ... the cause of registration cannot fail of accomplishment in the near future in Canada." The need for standards was added because it was thought that it was of "vital importance to the profession that there be uniformity of standards, that the training and registering of nurses be the same, fundamentally, in all parts of Canada." Support for these suggestions was reflected in the fact that by 1920, thirty-five associations of graduate nurses from across Canada had joined the national organization.[42] Occasionally an issue of The Canadian Nurse contained actual registration examinations that were provincially administered to foster continued support.[43]

Canadian nursing made considerable progress in its quest for professionalism during and after these two crises. In spite of their growing strength and self-confidence, hints of confusion began to appear when the reality of nursing practice encountered the professional ideological vision. Nurses in the private duty sector were concerned with working conditions and joined the nursing education debate.[44] Both private duty nurses and nursing educators agreed that ideally, independence and initiative should be encouraged in student nurses. The nurse educators, however, suggested that these attributes be used to encourage altruism, not efforts to improve the workplace. For many of them, real nursing was still mothering and they expressed concern that to drop the "heart" from nursing was to allow it to degenerate into a commonplace, utilitarian occupation that anyone could follow.[45]

These questions were elaborated on in a lengthy and detailed discussion of The Higher Aspect of Nursing published in 1919. The writer addressed the immorality that was negatively affecting "many beautiful and noble souls, with the loftiest ideals, who are striving to give the best of their lives to the cause of Humanity."[46] Nursing ideals such as these would stay with the profession for decades and would create considerable tension for nursing generally. However, the tension gave further impetus to the leaders of the profession to move to take control of the educational preparation of nurses. In this regard, any confusion was superseded by the fact that nursing education, at least in public health, was now offered within the walls of the university.

Given the events of this period, it is not surprising to note that physicians continued to be very much involved with nursing and their involvement was changing. Consequently, in 1919, Dr. Helen MacMurchy, a female physician and staunch friend of nursing, made a presentation to Toronto's Central Registry of Nurses. She addressed "The Future of the Nursing Profession." MacMurchy had been closely associated with nursing in Canada for a number of years and, as the first editor of The Canadian Nurse, her ideas were well received. MacMurchy identified a number of areas that required attention from Canadian nurses:

> First, a great and even greater number of nurses are needed ... And second, new developments of the work of trained nurses are always appearing ... The nursing profession has ... had no time ... to standardize its education, and obtain the necessary legislation to protect the public and enable the profession to do its best for the public. This must be done soon and as well as we can.[47]

MacMurchy elaborated on these points to address conditions of work in terms of financial remuneration and hours of work. Nursing in Canada had reached a new plateau and was now ready to move confidently towards improvements in these areas.

These years, 1914 to 1919 therefore, represent a period in which nurses were afforded the opportunity to begin to take control of their profession. The outbreak of the Spanish Flu and the poor physical health of veterans resulted in a new increased awareness of both issues. Nurses, particularly those who had volunteered overseas, along with the Canadian Red Cross Society were identified as the group that would be of the most value in this regard. The growing importance of science not only contributed to professionalism in nursing but also began to gradually erode the altruistic idealism in the Nightingale legacy. As noted in the Toronto General Hospital's <u>History</u>:

> 1920 was Nightingale Year in nursing history. In 1820 Florence Nightingale was born, and throughout the English speaking world nurses celebrated her centenary year, by emphasizing the amazing history of nursing. In seventy years a thoroughly adequate professional organization had been developed and remained – all the proof that could ever, in the past or in the future, be needed of the administrative talents of women.[48]

Therefore, in spite of the conservative lens through which women were viewed, nursing emerged as a strong force in Canadian health care delivery. This state of affairs coincided with two events that guaranteed successful results for nursing and was closely connected to the interactive relationship nurses maintained with their surrounding society. Nurses proved their value in the delivery of their services to the Canadian Expeditionary Forces during the War and faced another opportunity, during the influenza epidemic, to build on that well-deserved reputation. Taken together, these events afforded nursing two occasions to prove themselves and the worth of their services to Canadian society. Proof of their success lies in the support Canadians gave nursing leaders in initiating their campaign towards professionalism.

CHAPTER TWO NOTES

[1] Quoted in John Murray Gibbon & Mary S. Mathewson, Three Centuries of Canadian Nursing, (Toronto: MacMillan Company of Canada, 1947), p. 342.

[2] Helen K. Mussallem, "Nurses and Political Action" in B.Lasor & M.R.Elliott, eds., Issues in Canadian Nursing, (Scarborough: Prentice Hall, 1977), p. 158.

[3] M. Kathleen King, "The Development of University Nursing Education" in Mary Q. Innis, ed., Nursing Education in a Changing Society, (Toronto: University of Toronto Press, 1970), p. 69.

[4] Gibbon & Mathewson, Three Centuries, p. 296.

[5] The Leaf and the Lamp, p. 64.

[6] A Brief History, p. 40,41. At this, the Sixth General Meeting of the Canadian National Association of Trained Nurses, twenty-seven affiliated associations were represented by delegates.

[7] Agnes J. Macleod, "Military and Veteran Care Nursing," CN, Vol.51, No.3, March 1955, p. 214

[8] Robert Bothwell et al. Canada 1900-1945, (Toronto: University of Toronto Press, 1987), p. 158., p. 159.

[9] Anne E. Ross, Narrative of World War I Nursing Service, NAC, Mg 30, E446., p. 3.

[10] Apparently those nursing sisters who died in the torpedoed ship H.M.S. Llandovery Castle faced their attack calmly as noted in Kathryn Symonds Catterill compilation, "The Alumnae Association Incorporated of the Royal Victoria Hospital School for Nurses: 1896-1972," 1972, p. 11.

[11] Anne E. Ross, Narrative, p. 12.

[12] Ibid., p. 13.

[13] Ibid., p. 14.

[14] Ibid., p. 9.

[15] Gibbon & Mathewson, Three Centuries, p. 307.

[16] Ibid., pp. 302,307,308.

[17] D. Scollard, Hospital: A Portrait of Calgary General Hospital, (Calgary: Calgary General Hospital, 1981), p. 27.

[18] Janice P. Dickin-McGinnis, "The Impact of Epidemic Influenza: Canada, 1918-1919," in S.E.D. Shortt, ed., Medicine in Canadian Society: Historical Perspectives, (Montreal: McGill-Queen's University Press, 1981), p. 449, 124.

[19] Eileen Pettigrew, The Silent Enemy: Canada and the Deadly Flu of 1918, (Saskatoon: Western Producer Prairie Books, 1983), p. 6.

[20] Dr. Margaret Patterson, "Spanish Influenza: S.O.S. Lectures Nos. 1 and 2, to Young Lady Volunteers," The Toronto World, October 16, 1918, p. 10.

[21] D. Scollard, Hospital, p. 29.

[22] "Wanted, Volunteers!!," Ottawa Journal, October 16, 1918, p. 5.

[23] Daily Herald, November 2, 1918, p. 6.

[24] The Toronto World, October 26, 1918, p. 1.

[25] The Globe, October 11, 1918, p. 12.

[26] J.P. Dickin-McGinnis, "The Impact of Epidemic Influenza:," p.471.

[27] "Nurses," 1919, Victorian Order of Nurses, NAC, MG. 28, I 171, Vol.6, 6-2.

[28] Mitzi I.R. Montgomery, "The Legislative Healthscape of Canada: 1867-1975" in B.Lasor & M.R.Elliott, ed., Issues in Canadian Nursing, (Scarborough: Prentice Hall, 1977), pp. 132-134.

[29] Neil Sutherland, Children in English Canadian Society: Framing the Twentieth Century Consensus, (Toronto: University of Toronto Press, 1976), p. 39.

[30] Neil Sutherland, "School Children in the Public Health Movement, 1880-1914" in S.E.D.Shortt, ed., Medicine in Canadian Society: Historical Perspectives, (Montreal: McGill Queen's University Press, 1981), p. 363, 378.

[31] Theresa Christy, "A History of the Division of Nursing Education of Teacher's College, Columbia University, 1899-1944," Ph.D. Dissertation, University of Michigan, 1970, p. 80.

[32] A Brief History, p. 33.

[33] Ella Phillips Crandell, "The Nurse's Part in the Promotion of Public Health," CN, Vol.IX, No.7, July 1913, p. 444.

[34] A Brief History, p. 42.

[35] Lawrence, History, p. 37.

[36] Gibbon & Mathewson, Three Centuries, p. 332.

[37] A Brief History, p. 51.

[38] Geo. G.Nasmith, Chairman, Committee of the Canadian Red Cross Society, to Sir Robert A.Falconer, President, University of Toronto, March 15, 1920, UTA, A 73-0053.

[39] D.Scollard, Hospital, p. 32.

[40] "Injured," "License the Nursing Profession," The Globe, N.D., 1918, CNAA.

[41] Canadian National Association of Trained Nurses to The Globe, June 5, 1918, CNA Archival Correspondence, CNAA.

[42] A Brief History, pp. 22, 29, 23-54. BC.(5), AB.(3), Sask.(1), Man.(2), Ont.(19), PQ.(4), NS.(1).

[43] CN, Vol.XII, No.3, March 1916, pp. 134-137.

[44] M.Wolcraft, "The Editor's Letter Box," Trained Nurse and Hospital Review (TNHR), Vol.63, No.1, July 1919, p. 44.

[45] Annette Fisk, "Importance of Training Women for Private Duty Nursing," TNHR, Vol.64, No.1, January 1920, pp. 16-18., p. 17.

[46] Gertrude Harding, The Higher Aspect of Nursing, (Philadelphia: W.B. Saunders Company, 1919), pp. 10, 303. This text was found in the archives of the Civic Hospital in Ottawa.

[47] Helen MacMurchy, M.D. "The Future of the Nursing Profession," CN, Vol.XVI, No.2, February 1920, pp. 70-71.

[48] Lawrence, History, pp. 40-41.

Chapter Three

THE DILEMMA OF THE 1920S

The 1920s saw the establishment of public health nursing as an organized body. Advanced educational programs in public health nursing were established across the country and the need for this service was publicized. Nursing registration acts were in place in all the provinces by 1922. Therefore, the focus of the leadership activity in terms of professionalism during the twenties was the standardization and possible advancement of nursing education. Within this context, Canadian nurses continued their pursuit of professionalism but during these years, progress was unequal. Indeed, the irregularity that occurred in the progress of nursing resulted from the tension that was created by the desire of the nursing leaders to push for professionalism and the resistance on the part of the private duty nurses, who to a large degree, continued to cling to the old concept of nursing as a vocation. Despite the post-war public support for nursing, their pursuit of professionalism met with opposition from both the medical profession and the public. The ebb and flow of the success of nursing during this decade was also a reflection of the boom and bust economy that Canadians experienced throughout the twenties.

Two distinct groups of nurses organized themselves during the twenties; private duty nurses and public health nurses. Although all nurses concerned themselves with the health of the Canadian public, their actions were influenced by their unique role within the nursing community itself. Nursing leaders directed their energies towards the educational preparation of the nurse that would lend credibility to the occupation and culminate in professionalization. The private duty nurses were more concerned with the practical realities of nursing service and appropriate recognition of that service. Public health nurses, in many ways, addressed both the educational and service components of professionalism but also contributed to the tensions that materialized between the other two groups. Nursing was caught between the ideology of professionalism that demanded advanced educational preparation and the practical demands of nursing service. Not all nurses agreed with the educational goals of the nursing leaders. When nursing leaders were unable to arrive at a consensus with other nurses on this issue, they looked to the medical profession and the public at large for assistance only to discover that this strategy often added to their predicament.

At the outset of the decade, it was clear that the state supported the valuable role nurses now played in maintaining the health of Canadians. Indeed, the newly constituted Dominion Council of Health advised that the department initiate "a program of public education, a rapid expansion of hospital facilities ... registration of all available nurses, emergency medical training of volunteers, and registration of any voluntary home helpers to ensure the realization of this goal."[1] Furthermore, it was realized that during a disaster, the nurse was the key factor in both the prevention and spread of disease.[2] In spite of the growing trend of nursing towards professionalization, the state continued to emphasize nursing service as a noble, tender ministry provided by heroic women. Indeed, William Lyon Mackenzie King inscribed words to this effect on the Memorial to the Canadian Nurses in the Great War. Canadian nurses funded this memorial thus clearly demonstrating their support of this view. Furthermore, ideas such as these were articulated in poetic verse in The Canadian Nurse as well.[3] But, Ethel Johns, a prominent nurse in British Columbia, represented a departure from this traditional view. In 1920, before a joint meeting of the British Columbia Hospital Association and the Public Health Association she made an emphatic appeal for professional education for nurses when she protested:

> In Canada today any person or group of persons may assemble a number of sick persons under a roof and call that place a hospital. Further, they may offer to young women instruction in one of the most vital and difficult of arts. It would be reasonable to suppose that before so doing it would be necessary to assure some competent authority that conditions in that school were such as would insure the pupil competent instruction and proper living and working conditions. Such is not the case. The only point in which specific legislation exists in most of our provinces is that a certain number of beds – *beds*, mark you, *not patients*, must be available before a training school is established. And what is this minimum? In some provinces as high as twenty-five in others as low as five. No mention of qualified instructors, no restrictions as to hours of duty, no provision for teaching equipment – just beds and pupils.[4]

For Canadians, the difficulties and uncertainties of the twenties began with the dramatic shift to urban living. The census of 1921 documented that 50 percent of Canadians were urban dwellers. In order to support themselves and their families in the urban environment, women entered the labour force in increasing numbers and doubled their representation in both teaching and nursing. The mainstream feminist ideology of the day, "maternal feminism," allowed for and encouraged women to participate in work that suited their "unique biological qualities." Therefore, the pursuit of nursing ensured that each individual aspirant would remain within her "proper sphere." As one nurse who entered nursing at the time noted:

> At that time a young girl ... had two choices. She could go into nursing, that was alright. She could go into teaching,

67

that was alright. But if she went into be[ing] a secretary... that was not alright. What was respectable was teaching and nursing, those were the two respectable things ... it was well-looked upon, it was alright to go and be a nurse, it was very good.[5]

Nursing had become an acceptable pursuit for young women. As an occupation, it enabled them to combine a career with an appropriately feminine role.

These changes were accompanied by the emergence of a new definition of the role of the state constructed by the social scientific community. The practical demands of a post-war society contributed to the perception that there existed a need for state intervention for the sake of the potential of the individual on whose behalf the intervention was taking place. The passage of the Department of Health Act offers one example of the general acceptance of this ideology. The growing faith in medical science extended to the community of social scientists. These experts dictated what services were necessary and who was to design and administer those services. The 1920s witnessed spectacular growth in the numbers of social workers as paid professionals on the public payroll. As the decade progressed, numerous organizations of social workers sprang into existence. Further evidence of their professional status lay in their claim to the possession of a range of skills that verified their work as a scientific craft. This transformation of social work during the twenties into a secular profession corresponded with the general shift in orientation within Canadian society.[6] This shift was related to the increasing accessibility of Canadians to educational opportunities that affected their skill levels, literacy, attitudes, and values and further contributed to a secularization of society. The new professionals, however, wanted careers not sainthood. Furthermore, this escalating importance of expertise presented nursing with additional ammunition for its campaign towards professionalism.

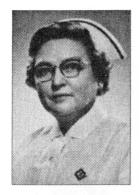

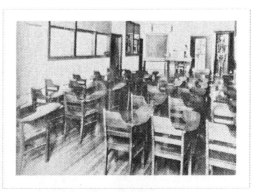

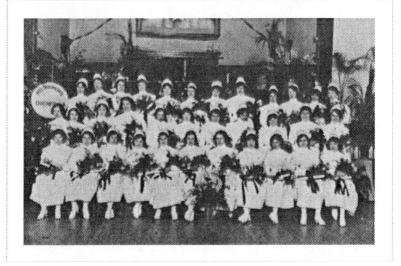

CLOCKWISE FROM TOP LEFT: Edith G. Young, Director of Nursing at the Ottawa Civic Hospital from 1946 to 1964. (Courtesy Ottawa Civic Hospital School of Nursing Alumnae) / Student nurses' classroom during the twenties. (Courtesy Ottawa Civic Hospital Alumnae) / Graduating class of 1924, Calgary General Hospital. (Courtesy Calgary General Hospital School of Nursing Alumnae)

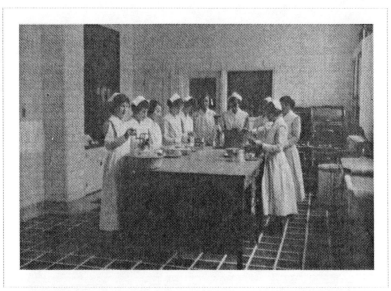

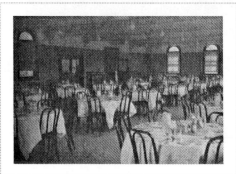

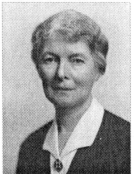

CLOCKWISE FROM TOP LEFT : Student nurses enjoying a class in the Diet Kitchen of the Ottawa Civic Hospital. / The Dining Room for the student nurses - a necessary part of the socialization process for the young women who entered nursing. (Both photos courtesy of the Ottawa Civic Hospital Alumnae) / Edith MacPherson-Dickson, CNA President 1920 - 22 (Courtesy Helen K. Mussallem Library).

The focus of Canadian nursing leaders was to bring to nursing a system of improved educational preparation. The tone was set early in the decade when Helen Randal, the current editor of The Canadian Nurse, urged nurses to subscribe to their national magazine because:

> If all nurses realized the power of the professional press, if properly used and the magazine read as it should be by every Canadian nurse wherever and whatever she is, then we would see a revival of the true spirit of nursing, and we could demonstrate that, as a profession, we were competent and willing to "clean house" whenever it was needed.[7]

Moreover, improved educational preparation programs would lead, as historian Heather MacDougall has argued, "to a set of behavioural prescriptions and understandings that are taught to new members as normal, correct, and appropriate ways to act and think."[8] Those women who entered nursing already shared a similar historical experience and social environment. Therefore, these improvements would build on the existing commonalities and promote unity within the group.

Another requirement of professionalism was government sanction. By 1922, all nine provinces had some form of Registration Act. Although the Acts differed provincially, most included educational requirements for admission to schools of nursing. In 1923, the Canadian National Association of Trained Nurses opened a national office in Winnipeg and employed Jean Scantlion Wilson as Executive Secretary. Provincial associations supported the national body in this appointment. As was noted in the Minutes taken at the Alberta Association of Registered Nurses convention in October 15, 1923:

> Possibly no one except the committees of the various provincial organizations realize how splendidly the secretary

appointed has co-operated with the various affiliated organizations in an endeavour to be helpful to them.[9]

The organization was given further reason to exist when Canadian nurses identified the need "for a bureau of information regarding positions in, and suitable applicants for, the various fields of nursing."[10] In 1923, the national body had the support of the provincial associations and as their representative, shortened its name to the Canadian Nurses Association. The next step was to improve the educational standards of nursing education. The first standard to be examined was the living and educational environments currently in operation in the various provinces. Therefore, the inspection of schools of nursing began on a provincial level.

The Ontario government appointed Alice Munn, Director of Nursing at Stratford General Hospital, as Director of the Department of Public Health in 1922. She was assigned the task of investigating the schools of nursing throughout the province with a view to closing those that did not adhere to the established criteria. In the first year she closed fifty-one nursing schools for a variety of reasons that included the lack of a library for the nursing students and double occupancy of one bed in the nurses' residence.[11]

Across the country in British Columbia, Helen Randal, from the Registered Nurses Association of British Columbia, performed a similar function. Randal could only make recommendations to the individual hospital boards but she did note improvements in "housing, working conditions and hours of work" following her visit. Indeed, she noted that some hospitals "appeared to understand that they had an obligation to provide an education."[12]

In 1922, Randal presented a paper to the national convention held in Edmonton that offered a complete overview of her work, obstacles encountered and the significance of her findings. She published her paper in The Canadian Nurse in order to assist other provincial associations in their pursuit of similar inspection tours.[13]

Nursing service and the exploitation of that service was often a part of the debate about nursing education, particularly when these issues encountered budgetary considerations. One such dialogue appeared in The Canadian Nurse:

> [Canadian Hospital] For instance, the X-ray machine could be installed in the Superintendent's office, if the Superintendent was an x-ray operator, which is sometimes the case. In most hospitals of the type under consideration, the Superintendent, a woman, is superintendent of nurses, instructor of nurses, operating-room nurse, x-ray operator, and general plant manager. Under such conditions facilities may be more readily combined, since but one facility is used at a time ...

> [Canadian Nurse] This arrangement certainly saves a room or two in the hospital but what of the Superintendent? More than that we, as an organization, made a real campaign to educate the public, and especially the part of it that acts as the Hospital Trustees or Boards of Governors of a hospital?[14]

This dialogue shows that nurses were now willing to argue their case against hospital exploitation of their services. Up to this point, nurses had willingly fulfilled all of the demands made of them. The reason for this was related to the Nightingale legacy of servitude as well as the hierarchical control supervisory nurses maintained over junior nurses. In many ways this conformity led to a versatility that then contributed to their indispensability in the hospital. However, nursing leaders' desire to move nursing away from the status of spiritual vocation necessitated an assertive stance in this regard. Therefore, the journal continued to call for improvements in nursing education. By the mid-1920s, the editor of The Canadian Nurse noted "the topic of Nursing Education is suffering from no neglect these days."[15] Unanimity of purpose however, was not always apparent.

The debate heated up considerably when a physician criticised any educational advancements because:

> to keep nurses learning new things every day without considerable intervals of routine will lead either to superficiality or mental break-down ... Her duty is to carry out accurately the instructions of the doctor as to the nursing of the patient; it is not her duty to assist in treating the patient. The argument that she should be in a position to understand all that the doctor is doing and ordering is fallacious.[16]

Jean E. Browne, president of the Canadian Nurses Association, criticised the "thoroughly trained automaton" that this physician promoted. She stated that nurses should insist on thinking for themselves so as to offer "intelligent cooperation" to the physician rather than "blind obedience." Further to this, since an "alert mind is a prime requisite for such a nurse," an improved educational curriculum was necessary.[17]

In 1928, nursing leaders linked the need for an improved education to the advances that had been made in the science of medicine. The benefits that would be realized by all of the parties involved were key to the discussion. It was understood to be of primary importance that the benefits be identified, given the fact that "the public must pay for nursing science."[18] In other words, nurses were asking for public funds to support nursing education so that schools of nursing would be financially independent educational institutions. In this way, the exploitation of student nurses would disappear and the students would acquire a standardized professional education rather than vocational apprenticeship training.

In June, 1927, the Canadian Nurses Association, in cooperation with the Canadian Medical Association and the provincial hospital associations met and struck a committee to investigate "the nursing problem." This "Study Committee" consisted of three nurses, three physicians, one layperson, and was chaired by Dr. G. Stewart Cameron, Chairman of the Canadian Medical Association's Committee on Nursing. The Canadian Nurses Association and the Canadian Medical Association would share expenses incurred by the Committee. The nurses were Jean Gunn from the Toronto General Hospital, Kathleen Russell, a public health nurse in Toronto and Jean Browne from the Canadian Red Cross. The problem areas that these three nurses identified were supply and demand, nursing and the public, hospital needs of nursing, private duty nurses and the medical profession, the nurse, nursing education, and a study of the professional registration acts in Canada.[19] The report proposed to be comprehensive.

In 1929, the Committee would continue this investigation under the direction of George M. Weir, a professor at the University of British Columbia. The investigation became known as the Survey of Nursing Education in Canada or, "The Weir Report," and the general aims were:

> To assist the nursing profession by crystallizing its problems and by defining and elevating its status.

> To render more effective assistance to the medical profession in its great service to suffering humanity.

> Primarily to promote the interests and well-being of the patient and of the public.[20]

Weir set out his plan clearly in The Canadian Nurse and requested the wholehearted cooperation and support of both nurses and physicians for this detailed survey. The editor of The Canadian Nurse encouraged all nurses to "adopt the slogan 'Survey First'" and gave further justification for the basic need for such an examination of nursing in Canada. In this way the support of Canadian nurses was enlisted and indeed, received for what would later be a very lengthy and complex report, published in 1932. It was hoped that an investigation such as this would lend further support to nursing's claim to professionalism.

Nursing education was a topic that interested not only nurses, physicians, and hospitals but individual Canadians as well. For example, in his will, Harry Judson Crowe, a Torontonian born in Halifax, gave financial support to advanced nursing education. Crowe had spent a significant portion of his life in hospital and had noted the arduous work entailed in nursing, the lack of leisure time, and the fact that nurses were often weakened physically in the course of their career. He concluded that all of this resulted in a nurse who was often destitute of funds. Given the singular importance of the nurse in the community, this gentleman felt that "the nursing profession should receive greater recognition and encouragement." To this end he left one-third of his residuary estate as follows:

> The bequest is to take the form of annual scholarships to the value of six hundred dollars each for an approximate period of ten years, these scholarships being awarded to a graduate from the largest public inter-denominational hospital, in the largest city by way of population of each of the provinces of Canada, and also the Dominion of Newfoundland. In Ontario the Toronto General Hospital is the designated hospital, and in Nova Scotia the Victoria General Hospital of Halifax. It is further stated that this last mentioned hospital should receive each year double the number of scholarships awarded to any of the other hospitals in other provinces.[21]

The scholarships were to support nurses in pursuit of post-graduate nursing education currently available at seven universities across Canada. Bequests such as this supported nursing aspirations for professionalism, particularly with regard to public health nursing. Indeed, this group of nurses was the first to be accorded any degree of professional recognition.

Public health nurses achieved formal organization early in the 1920s and were a privileged group in that they had popular and political support through the Canadian Red Cross Society. Clearly, the earlier flu epidemic had contributed to the support given to public health by the Canadian Red Cross Society. This recognition gave public health nursing professional legitimacy that was advanced further by their university educational preparation.

The first class in public health nursing graduated from Dalhousie University in 1920 and graduates followed these fifteen women quickly from universities across Canada. The need for this type of nursing grew with the clarification and development of the definition of 'public health'. Public health nurses themselves clearly heightened the professional image of their group in discourses regarding their service. For them:

> Public health is the science and the art of preventing disease, prolonging life and promoting physical health and efficiency through organized community efforts for the sanitation of the environment, the education of the individual in principles of personal hygiene, the organization of medical and nursing service for the early diagnosis and preventive treatment of disease, and the development of the social machinery which will insure to every individual in the community a standard of living adequate for the maintenance of health.[22]

The nurse was the contact person in this process and therefore had a monumental mediatory role in the delivery of professional public health services.

Nursing skill became a valued commodity to the public and public health nursing achieved even greater prominence. The Ladies' Home Journal popularized and publicized this career by describing public health nurses as:

> capable, intelligent women, with the training which makes them able to contribute to society something which society wants, have waiting for them well-paid, interesting positions, opportunities to use their own initiative, to see the influence of their health-bringing message upon tired

mothers, overworked fathers, undernourished or unintentionally neglected children; in fact, to become a real part of the progress which is daily making America a safer and happier place to live in.[23]

The public health nurse was first of all a teacher acting as a community agency. She worked in the school and in the home with the entire family and was viewed as the single most important factor "in the creation of an environment conducive to healthy living."[24] There were three aspects to her work; educative, preventive, and curative. Furthermore, the public health nurse was an agent:

> working among the people in their homes teaching the value of modern medicine, advising, stimulating and helping people to have medical attention and building up an ideal of health. The public health nurse is the interpreter, the messenger, this teacher in the home.[25]

The need for prevention and teaching in the home was, of course, associated with the rapid spread of tuberculosis and the prevention of disease in children.[26] However, as the role of the public health nurse expanded, her service gained in professional status.

During these early years, growth was slow and the public health nursing committee looked to the Canadian Nurses Association to assist in strengthening the public health nursing group. With the cooperation of the Victorian Order of Nurses and financial support of the Canadian Red Cross Society, the educational preparation of public health nurses advanced. This gave the public health nurses the confidence needed and they began to organize their group to promote their particular nursing service as an indispensable public service. Indeed, the Public Health Nursing section of the Canadian National Association of Trained Nurses was formed in 1921 and the programme of the Eleventh General Meeting of this organization was devoted to public health nursing concerns. Furthermore, the unique role played by the public health nurse in the community allowed her to function as an independent practitioner of nursing. These nurses were viewed from within and without as professionals and as opportunities in their field expanded, active recruitment of nursing students occurred.[27] The medical profession, often grudgingly, relied upon the services of public health nurses in both rural and urban areas.

As the service became more popular, more nurses were needed and public health nursing was promoted within the ranks of nursing itself. The popularity of the work is reflected in their growing numbers. By 1922, there were one thousand public health nurses in Canada working independently within, and responsible to, a particular community. A further reflection of the important role given to public health nursing was that an entire section at the 1929 meeting of the International Council of Nurses in Montreal was devoted to that topic.[28] One paper entitled, "Rural Nursing from the Viewpoint of a Public Health Nurse" was presented by Elizabeth Smellie, a leader in public health nursing in Canada. Taken together, all of these events point to not only rapid growth in public health nursing, but acceleration in their professional recognition.

In spite of the apparent success of public health nurses, the pursuit of professionalism continued to be obstructed by the traditional view that associated nursing with motherhood. Indeed, in 1929, the The Canadian Nurse published an article which described the practice of nursing as an activity that occurred "wherever there is life to be tended, nourished or nursed, whether the life be yet unborn, or new-born, or senile, or ill, there is the field for womanhood exercising its great function of foster motherhood."[29] The competing ideals of professionalism and mothering kept everyone confused in this period. The terminology associated with nursing was usually borrowed from the nomenclature that surrounded the 'family'. Nursing leaders attempted to rationalize this situation through professional education but only brought further confusion to the situation.

Consequently, this intellectual dilemma trickled down into the realm of the private duty nurses.

Private duty nurses viewed their work as the highest form of nursing due to the spirit of devotion and self-sacrifice that it involved. Most graduate nurses were employed outside of the hospital in the homes of their patients. These nurses discussed professionalism chiefly in terms of service, not educational preparation, but did consider themselves to be equal partners with the other branches of the profession. Having accepted their professional status, however, some private duty nurses believed that satisfactory compensation was to be found in the reward of a satisfied mind.[30]

The service ideal was a given. Indeed, it was noted that, "the public demands a nurse who is well trained, strong in body and calm in mind, with an inexhaustible supply of cheerful common sense."[31] Furthermore, obituaries praised qualities such as humility and deference as attributes to be admired in a nurse. One example was the obituary that described the characteristics of an ideal, albeit deceased, nurse who "was modest and retiring almost to a fault, never seeking praise for herself, but always so ready to give praise, when due, to others."[32] In this way, humility and self-sacrifice were promoted as essential if one aspired to be a professional nurse.

The nursing service ideal was closely connected to nursing ethics, which was always cause for invoking religion and spirituality. This is not surprising given that most Canadians continued to be very much taken up with religion and the new and evolving social order. Words such as obedience, deference, loyalty, and honour were usually associated with what nurses termed the "professional nurse."[33] One nurse recommended that daily reading of the "Book" would provide infallible guidance to one's nursing practice.[34] If the nurse incorporated all of these elements into her daily work, she would then be able to maintain the high standards of the profession. The "perfect nurse" was described repeatedly in The Canadian Nurse as one who participated in a career that was often viewed as a professional 'calling':

> No calling, however, offers a greater opportunity for service of the higher type than does the nursing profession, which embodies in its purposes everything we regard as lofty and altruistic. Endowed as they are by nature and by training with moral and physical qualities of the highest order; and with their feminine sympathies attuned to the cries of the afflicted, to whom among ourselves, should we look for leadership in our itinerary toward the light, if not to our nurses?[35]

Although written by a physician, this stereotypical description of a nurse continued to depict the ideal nurse as a paragon of virtue. These ideas would have been familiar to the graduate nurses of the day because the pure joy of service was the chief reward to be found in nursing. Service was key to the justification of the ordinary nurse's very existence and striving for this ideal was the closest that private duty nurses came to any discussion of professionalism.

The average graduate nurse, whether in private duty or in institutional nursing, was too busy caring for her patients and herself to become involved in any of the larger issues of professionalism. This was apparent in the following reflection of Isabel Irvine, a 1925 graduate of The Lady Stanley Institute for Trained Nurses:

> It was the first case I had in a private home and I was there for six weeks. For the first two weeks there were two nurses; one for days and I was on nights. We were on twelve hour shifts and included our meals. As he improved I was put on a 24 hour shift which paid six dollars per shift. That was the going wage and if you didn't take it you were unemployed because there was an abundance of nurses. I had two hours

off in the afternoon and slept on a single bed just outside the patient's door if he needed a nurse at night.[36]

Another example of the need for the nurse's energies to be directed toward the work-at-hand is apparent in Edith Young's (a 1922 graduate) description of one of her early cases:

> I will describe ... a pneumonia patient in the country. After five days working twenty-four hours per day with a few snoozes on the chair, I was relieved for four hours sleep. The patient did not recover. I was called upon to prepare her for the coffin including dressing her and curling her hair. She was then placed on a broad board supported by two chairs awaiting the coffin, which was transported to the home by the family in a wagon drawn by two horses.[37]

This type of experience was true for most graduate nurses. One nurse in rural Alberta was far more committed to nursing her patient following a thyroidectomy or the patient recovering from a broken back than engaging in any of the debates concerning issues of professionalism. Indeed another nurse, a 1927 graduate from the Calgary General Hospital, stated quite matter-of-factly that her only concern involved her duties as Night Supervisor and that she was completely unaware of issues surrounding professionalism.[38]

These anecdotes offer further evidence that the typical graduate nurse was only concerned with the delivery of nursing service. In this way, the vast majority of nurses active in the home or the institution were taking care of the business of nursing on a practical level. Clearly, these nurses were in agreement regarding the function and purpose of nursing. Their practical perspective, however, was at odds with that of their nursing leaders and that of the public health nurses.

Dissension first appeared in a discussion between the private duty nurses and Ethel Johns, Director of Nursing at the Vancouver General Hospital. Johns addressed the future of private duty nursing and the inability of the nurse involved in that line of work to gain satisfaction in her work in the first year of practice. She attributed the dissatisfaction to the low wages and lengthy shifts but she also pointed out that there was some discontent with private duty nurses amongst the medical profession and the public in general. She challenged the private duty nurses to organize themselves, broaden their knowledge, and take charge of the situation. One private duty nurse took exception to these observations and wrote a letter to <u>The Canadian Nurse</u> expressing her disgruntlement. This nurse challenged the superintendents to "clean their own steps" before intruding into the affairs of other nursing groups. The writer was also critical of the fact that there was very little discussion of the topic of nursing at the Canadian Nurses Association conventions and that perhaps this situation might be rectified at the next meeting. Although the letter was unsigned, its publication indicates an acknowledgment of the general feeling of unrest that was apparent among this group of nurses.[39]

Criticism such as this contributed to the ongoing rumblings of discontent among the private duty nurses. They were accused by nursing leaders of silence and ineffectiveness regarding their profession. They replied with the following justification:

> Long hours of labour of the most exacting and exhausting nature are disastrous to clearness and originality of thought, and the absolute lack of time for much-needed recreation, proper reading, religious exercises and social intercourse, which privileges the other branches of the profession enjoy to a far greater extent than does the private duty nurse, are not calculated to be productive of any very valuable or enlightening assistance from a body so handicapped.[40]

The writer suggested that a shorter workday would definitely reduce the fatigue of the nurse and since the private duty nurses made up the largest group in the profession, consultation with, or acknowledgment of their situation, from the professional

83

organizations would be helpful. She noted the escalating tensions within nursing and called for united and harmonious cooperation.

The Private Duty Committee, established in 1921, decided to investigate the improvement of working conditions for nurses, in particular, the need for insurance and pensions.[41] By 1927, some private duty nurses carried insurance against accident and sickness and some even had Endowment Insurance but wondered if they would live to receive the final amount.[42] The national organization responded with the approval of a resolution in 1924 that recommended Nursing Superintendents across Canada experiment with a ten-hour day for nurses working in the hospitals.[43] As a recommendation, it represented only token support of the plight of the private duty nurse and did not address the fundamental survival issues associated with insurance and pensions.

Wages were low and varied from place to place but compared favourably with that of a teacher if the nurse worked 240 days in the year and was actually paid. However, the expenses incurred by a nurse were much higher than that of a teacher. Expenses such as laundry, maintenance of a work and social wardrobe plus the expense of travel contributed to a significant financial burden. This topic was given elaborate coverage in a presentation to the 1922 meeting of the Canadian National Association of Trained Nurses in Edmonton. The speaker, a physician of forty years, ruminated on "what is then the recompense of the labours of this profession and why do women take it up?." His answer:

> from one who has witnessed the rise and progress of the trained nurse's calling is the sense of duty nobly done to the glory of God and the service of your fellow man - the complete fulfillment of 'The Law', and, combined with an humble walk through life, all that the Lord requires of man.[44]

The practical concerns of the graduate nurse were rarely given serious consideration thus adding to their frustration. Seldom did the nursing leadership make any concrete suggestions, which in turn, contributed to a growing division within nursing. This division only magnified the tensions between the two views: nursing as a vocation versus nursing as a profession.

Public health nurses, on the other hand, faced attacks on two fronts, from their nursing colleagues and their medical superiors. Members of their own profession viewed them with contempt because they worked with the "public." The medical profession objected to them because they believed that the public health nurses were offering medical advice without a medical license to practice and thus undermined the faith of the patient and the family in the physician.[45] In spite of this untenable position, the fact that public health nurses often worked in isolated areas considered undesirable by physicians contributed to the view that their role was necessary and, therefore, tolerable. However, their geographic isolation also removed them from the epicentre of most debates.

Activities directed towards the attainment of professionalism were prominent in the development of all three groups of nurses. Although they appeared to be united in this goal, tensions became visible and brought considerable stress to bear on Canadian nursing. Elizabeth Smellie noted the mounting interdisciplinary tensions that appeared at the time. She commented that all nursing specialties were linked through the national organization and that the apparent rivalry and competition was understandable given the individual appeal of each nursing specialty. She encouraged nurses, however, to be aware of their interdependence through the national body and "to advance slowly along sound lines."[46]

One issue of contention was midwifery. It not only divided nurses but brought the nurses' loyalty to the medical profession into question. Competition between physicians and midwives was particularly noticeable in the delivery of health services to new Canadians from Central Europe. A Winnipeg hospital noted that:

> We quote the opinion of our leading doctors in the obstetrical department. 'The majority, at least 80%, of the Ukrainian women in Winnipeg, avail themselves of the services of qualified doctors and nurses at childbirth. In the course of the last ten years there has been a most noticeable decline in the demand for midwives among all Central European women at childbirth. At this rate, in the course of a few more years the midwife will be a thing of the past.[47]

Nurses were committed to maternal and childcare but refused to support the work of the midwife in rural Canada because of the apparent encroachment of the service into medical territory.

As early as 1919, trained nurses were allowed to assist in the delivery of babies in rural Alberta if a physician was not available. But, in 1923, the Alberta Association for Graduate Nurses passed a resolution against the practice of midwifery with the recommendation that "properly qualified medical men be attached to these districts."[48] Further support for this resolution was offered in a recommendation made by the Canadian Nurses Association that incentive pay be offered to physicians to practice in rural areas, that small outposts with a registered nurse in charge be established, and that an efficient transportation service be created and maintained.[49]

However, during the twenties, the situation became more difficult. In 1925, nurses supported the following Canadian Nurses Association resolution:

> Whereas, the membership in the CNA is strictly conditioned by professional standards, and the organization exists for the maintenance and elevation of these standards, and Whereas the CNA does not function apart from its federated units, it is not feasible to be affiliated with National Societies which do not conform to a similar plan of organization: Therefore

be it Resolved that the Association withdraw from the National Council of Women, the Social Service of Canada, and the Child Welfare Council of Canada.[50]

In other words, the professional organization that represented all Canadian nurses withdrew its affiliation from organizations such as the National Council of Women that supported the independent practice of midwifery. Nurses were torn between their need for support from the medical profession and their commitment to maternal and childcare.

The National Council of Women and their local affiliates shared the latter concern, particularly in rural Canada where women were at greater risk because obstetrical care was not easily accessible. The National Council of Women promoted the value of midwives in rural Canada but the professional organization that represented nursing chose to support the side taken by medicine. The decision made by nursing leaders to side with the medical profession in this debate is a clear manifestation of the tensions that existed within nursing. The practice of midwifery supported the independence associated with professionalism while the views of the medical profession promoted the subservience of nursing linked to the ideology of a vocation. Nonetheless, midwifery training programs continued at the local level but the Canadian Nurses Association appeared to ignore their existence. For example, Grace Agar graduated from a six-month midwifery training program at the Scottish Nursing Home in Calgary, in 1923, and proceeded to deliver babies across the prairies. The Canadian Nurses Association maintained a distant relationship with the National Council of Women because of this issue.[51]

Isolation and division clearly characterized nursing at this time but one area in which nurses joined all Canadians was in the maintenance and preservation of a white Anglo-Saxon Canada. Since all aspects of nursing are closely connected to hygiene, it is not surprising to learn that nurses were also concerned with mental hygiene, social hygiene, and mental illness. To date, the participation of nurses in this area has been given little attention by researchers but their close association with hygienic ventures necessitated their involvement. To this end, articles published in The Canadian Nurse addressed the sexual attitudes of nurses. It was generally agreed that sex was at the root of a great number of the ills from which the world was suffering – ills that nurses also combated.[52] One such ill was masturbation, which was closely linked to insane, criminal, or anti-social behaviour.

The public health nurse also addressed public hygiene in that she often worked with children and thus had the opportunity to identify those commonly referred to as idiot, or feeble-minded, children. The appearance of these children in a family was usually attributed to a history of insanity, poor environment, or poor hygiene on the part of the mother. The language of eugenics also appeared in articles discussing the type of young woman that should be accepted into a training school. Physical and intellectual defects not desirable to nursing were identified but the emphasis was on the worthiness of the prospective student for the profession.[53] The ease with which nursing made use of the vocabulary of eugenics reflects the interactive role nursing enjoyed with society at the time. For example, The Canadian Nurse published an article in 1929 entitled "Eliminating the Unfit from the School of Nursing." This interaction is especially exemplified in the role played by the public health nurse.

The services of a public health nurse might be viewed as a "Canadianizing" influence on the European immigrants. Health education and prevention of disease in this population contributed to the perception that the nurse acted as an agent of socialization. As one public health nurse wrote: "I have tried everything as perfectly as possible under the circumstances, and also to explain to them just why we think our way better than theirs."[54] The medical profession expressed their eugenics concerns in The Canadian Nurse. Nurses provided a fertile field for these ideas as most were white Anglo-Saxon protestants.

Their interest revolved around the fear that the standard of living might be lowered by the admission into Canadian society of immigrants who appeared to be defective in some way. The preferred way for a new Canadian to arrive in Canada was "in a cradle in a Canadian home." To this end, the physicians promoted "selective immigration."[55] These views were in keeping with much of Canadian society. Indeed, the earlier wave of immigration was stopped in 1930 when the newly elected Conservative government erected barriers to end it. The Depression added fuel to these early eugenics fears and public health nurses, in particular, later joined in support of the rhetoric. The support nurses gave to eugenics mirrored the assent of Canadian society in general and demonstrates the integral role nursing played in these social developments. Nonetheless, despite the support nurses gave the medical profession, their efforts did not result in reciprocity.

Opposition by physicians to advanced nursing education was considerable. E. Stanley Ryerson, a physician on the Medical Faculty of the University of Toronto, presented a paper at the meeting of the International Council of Nurses held in 1929, in Montreal. His paper, entitled, "The Preparation of a Curriculum" for a nursing educational program stated his position clearly:

> If the educational and academic instruction becomes the predominant feature of the course in the first place, both the personal and practical features suffer in consequence of being subsidiary with the result that the nurse is incompetent to perform her necessary functions: in the second, by gaining too great a scientific knowledge of diseases, the nurse has a tendency to become too professional in her attitude to the detriment of her services in a nursing capacity.[56]

Ryerson did suggest that a balanced approach to the practical, educational, and academic instruction be taken but reflected his medical bias in the fact that he limited the information that nurses should have of diseases to "prominent symptoms and signs and the explanation of their presence." Only medical students should learn about the etiology, pathology, symptomology, diagnosis, prognosis and treatment. For Ryerson, the purpose of a nursing educational program was to produce "a better and more cultured woman."[57] This goal suggests that Ryerson applied to nursing students the principles of public health: that of sanitizing, polishing and grooming.

Indeed, opposition from the medical profession greeted all proposals for advanced educational preparation for nurses. One physician pointed out that brains were not of primary importance in a nurse but rather her natural ability, because a good nurse was born and not made.[58] It was always emphasized that a good nurse was a good woman and that the necessary requisites were health, intelligence and a good conscience. Furthermore, "the training of a nurse includes two distinct parts: first, practical training in the care of the sick and prevention of disease; second, careful education in regard to her conduct."[59]

Physicians repeatedly stressed the importance of the practical side of nursing education. Indeed, "faith and hope" were more important than any lectures in psychology. Writers in the medical journal, Canada Lancet and Practitioner, suggested that every local medical society appoint a committee to investigate nursing education in their area and the national medical body would collect and study the data in order to make suggestions to the nursing profession regarding any improvements that might be made.[60]

Physicians also identified a number of problems associated with nursing. Articles were written about the talkative nurse, the bossy nurse, the lazy nurse, the over-sympathetic nurse and the undependable variety, all of whom would not be called upon for nursing service in the home.[61] The point to be made was the need for the approval of the physician if nurses wanted employment thus reflecting strong elements of dependency in the nurse-physician relationship. As another physician noted, "the private duty nurse must be loyal to the physician in charge of the case she is nursing ... She must be ready to respond to any call, if she registers for general duty."[62]

The dependent relationship nurses maintained with physicians contributed to the ongoing dilemma that confronted all nurses. Subservience limited their progress towards professionalism because approval from the medical profession was necessary before any advances could be made. Often this approval carried with it interference, usually unsolicited. Indeed, loyalty to the physician not only dictated developments in nursing but often also caused considerable division among nurses themselves.

The ideal professional nurse envisioned by nursing leaders was completely at odds with the ideal nurse envisioned by the medical profession and that contributed further to the tension and confusion within nursing. Physicians viewed the ideal nurse as a perfect woman who was intelligent, trustworthy, loyal, strong, courageous, patient, sympathetic, kindly, tactful and most importantly, looked to the physician for direction. Moreover, one other quality that was needed in this, a woman's natural vocation, was that of a strong body.[63] It was also noted that the ideal nurse had an innately pure mind and was accorded respect, adoration and love from her family and friends. Further to this, she loyally and respectfully carried out the wishes of the physician and specifically did not cause any trouble.[64]

One such ideal nurse was Sarah Edith Young, Lady Superintendent of the Training School for Nurses at the Montreal General Hospital, because "she possessed in marked degree those essential qualities of heart and mind of the ideal nurse and above all she was a good woman, whose influence was always felt by everyone who served with her."[65] Nursing leaders hoped that improvements in nursing education would initiate attitudinal changes among physicians, nurses and Canadians and thus establish nursing as a profession. To this end, their pursuit of standards in nursing education looked promising with the commencement of activities related to the eventual publication of the <u>Survey of Nursing Education in Canada</u>.[66]

Division and dissension within nursing contributed to the dilemma that faced Canadian nurses during the twenties, but created confusion for Canadians as well. The public expected missionary service from the nurse and expressed shock and disappointment when this expectation was not realized. The post-war view was that these young women had consecrated their lives to the service of the world's sufferers in the battle against dirt, disease, misery, and death. Indeed, one writer observed:

> I think we may safely say that the nurse who goes out in a spirit of unselfish devotion in peace or in war, in the homeland or in distant heathen lands beyond the sea to relieve the distressed, is following more closely than most of us the mind and the example of the Master.[67]

Therefore, missionary zeal accompanied most memories of nurses' experiences during World War I. Fond reflections noted that the nurses remained cool, alert and confident in the face of all of the wartime dangers. The aid and comfort the nurse offered to the wounded was equated with a clay vessel that was without flaw and could withstand heat and frost to "hold cool water for parched lips."[68]

Nurses were expected to be altruistic and therefore treated their patients as both a mother and a lover would. Indeed, in the purest form of altruism, the nurse dealt with ungrateful patients by offering them patience and kindness.[69] Altruism did not negate intelligence. Indeed, a young woman pursuing nursing education would be in a position to pursue lucrative work in a number of areas that included hospital nursing, school nursing, and rural nursing. According to an assistant director of nursing, dignity and responsibility was associated with many nursing positions, however, women in nursing had to have "the ability to take pains and the tireless, selfless will to be of service."[70] Indeed, a young woman pursuing nursing education would join a group of:

> capable, intelligent women, with the training which makes them able to contribute to society something which society wants, have waiting for them well-paid, interesting positions, opportunities to use their own initiative, to see the influence of their health-bringing message upon tired mothers, over-worked fathers, undernourished or unintentionally neglected children; in fact, to become a real part of the progress which is daily making America a safer and happier place to live in.

In this way the altruistic ideal was joined with the practical demands of nursing that elevated the nurse to being viewed as the epitome of selfless service.

Some patients, however, challenged this ideal with an opposing view. Often a private duty nurse in the home provoked the following reaction:

> If only they would do their duty a little better everything would be all right ... I haven't had to have one in my house for years, thank God ... I had to have a nurse last winter, and I sent for her in fear and trembling – I had heard such dreadful things. But she was a real joy. She did not even want to take two hours off ... Of course, there are nurses and nurses; but most of them are ... too horribly professional.[71]

Even in the hospital patients felt victimized. One individual who had been a patient in hospital for thirty-two months felt that he was a victim in a conspiracy while hospitalized. By this he meant that his very presence was an inconvenient nuisance to the nurse's desire to maintain a neat, tidy and efficient hospital.[72] Similarly, patients receiving nursing care in the home felt themselves to be overwhelmed by the nurse when she took command of their home because she appeared not to consider the needs and feelings of the family. A perfect nurse was one who was radiantly clean and wholesomely healthy, however, this nurse was the exception, not the rule. According to some patients who attended a symposium addressing this issue nurses were often insensitive, sloppy, lacked compassion, amusing and boring.[73]

Generally, however, nurses were regarded as promoters of cleanliness. This image of the nurse appeared regularly in advertisements associated with hygienic products. As an agent of hygiene, the nurse recommended products linked to nutrition, feminine hygiene, soaps, bathroom tissue, antiseptic solutions, toothpaste, soft drinks, facial creams and even life insurance.[74] General opinion maintained that nurses held an intense dislike for dirt and untidiness. Indeed, at the Toronto General Hospital, the Nursing Sister in Charge of a ward would not allow a "Vocational Officer" to install his accoutrements in her ward unless they were stored in a metal locker that harmonized esthetically with the other hospital furniture.[75] The emphasis was always on the wisdom of the nurse regarding the overwhelming importance of cleanliness. The nurse was viewed as an expert in this field and her image was of significant value in the successful marketing of hygienic products. Therefore, in spite of the mixed messages and related confusion that existed among nurses and society about nursing, society did acknowledge the nurse to be an expert in public hygiene.

Developments towards professionalism in Canadian nursing were uneven during the 1920s. Part of this unevenness can be attributed to the fact that nursing service increased in significance therefore, the need for the service grew proportionately. This growth resulted in the emergence of three formal groups of nurses: those in leadership, those at the bedside, and those working in public health. Nursing leaders concentrated on the pursuit of professionalism through legislation, organization, and advancing and standardizing nursing education. They obtained some success in that their endeavours culminated in the creation of a committee to investigate nursing education. However, nursing leaders failed to retain the unified support of the rapidly expanding numbers in nursing. Although the professional ideology promoted by the leaders received support from public health nurses, it did not transfer easily to the practical demands made of the nurse at the bedside. This division contributed to dissension within nursing that then gave rise to vulnerability within the group when it encountered opposition from the medical profession. Taken together, these circumstances created a dilemma for nursing and the community for whom they cared. Rather than submit to the confusion swirling within and around them, nursing leaders became proactive and together with the Canadian Medical Association and the Canadian Hospital Council the Association initiated an investigation into the "nursing problem" of the twenties, thus tenaciously pursuing their professional goal to standardize and then advance, nursing education.

CHAPTER THREE NOTES

[1] Janice Dickin McGinnis, "The Impact of Epidemic Influenza Canada, 1918-1919," p. 472.

[2] "Nursing in Disasters," CN. Vol. XVIII, No.1, January 1922, p. 9.

[3] "Recipe for Making a Good Nurse," CN, Vol. XVII, No.5, May 1921, p. 299, and "A Little of Everything," CN, Vol. XVIII, No.4, April 1922, p. 210.

[4] Quoted in Valerie Knowles, Leaving with a Rose: A History of the Ottawa Civic Hospital School of Nursing, (Ottawa: Ottawa Civic Hospital School of Nursing Alumnae Association, 1981), p. 33.

[5] Alice Girard - Videotaped interview, August, 1988, CNA President 1958-1960, retired Dean of the Faculty of Nursing at McGill University at Montreal.

[6] Doug Owram, The Government Generation: Canadian Intellectuals and the State 1900-1945, (Toronto: University of Toronto Press, 1986), p. 117-132.

[7] Helen Randal, "Annual Report of "The Canadian Nurse and Hospital Review," CN, Vol. XVIII, No.8, August 1922, p. 480.

[8] Heather MacDougall, Activists and Advocates, p. 51.

[9] "Minutes of the 7th Annual Convention," October 15, 1923, p. 5, Alberta Association of Registered Nurses Archives (AARNA), Edmonton, Alberta.

[10] Alberta Association of Graduate Nurses, "Official Minutes - Council," January 20, 1922, Vol.1, p. 131, AARNA.

[11] Videotaped interview in 1988 with Dorothy Riddell, Miss Munn's colleague. Riddell retired from the Ontario Department of Health in the sixties.

[12] Jo Ann Whittaker, "The Search for Legitimacy: Nurses' Registration in British Columbia, 1913-1935" in Barbara K. Latham & Roberta J. Pazdro, eds., Not Just Pin Money, (Victoria: Camosun College, 1984), p. 320.

[13] Helen Randal, "Inspection of Training Schools in British Columbia," CN, Vol. XIX, No.2, February 1923, p. 79-83.

[14] Helen Randal, "Editorial," CN, Vol. XIX, No.10, October 1923, p. 594.

[15] "Editorials," CN, Vol. XXI, No.4, April 1925, p. 177.

[16] "The Training of Nurses," CN, Vol. XXI, No.2, February 1925, pp. 81,82.

[17] Ibid., pp. 83, 84.

[18] Marion Lindeburgh et al, "The Organization of Community Interest in Nursing Education," CN, Vol. XXIV, No.9, September 1928, p. 464.

[19] "The Conference on Nursing," CN, Vol. XXIII, No.7, July 1927, pp. 364-366.

[20] Dr. George M. Weir, "Survey of Nursing Education in Canada," CN, Vol. XXV, No.11, November 1929, pp. 653,654.

[21] "A Gift to Nursing Education," CN, Vol. XXV, No.11, November 1929, p. 675.

[22] "Public Health Nursing Department," CN, Vol. XVIII, No.7, July 1922, p. 403.

[23] Ella Phillips Crandall, "Do I want my Daughter to Be a Nurse?," The Ladies' Home Journal, June 1920, p. 99.

[24] W.J. Bell, "The Public Health Nurse," CN, Vol. XIX, No.10, October 1923, pp. 601-605.

[25] Elizabeth G. Fox, "The Role of the Public Health Nurse," CN, Vol. XXIII, No.2, February 1927, pp. 72-75.

[26] David A. Stewart, "The Sanitorium, A University," CN, Vol. XXIII, No.5, May 1927, pp. 239-240; C. Wace, "Queen Alexandra Solarium," pp. 241-243; Meta Hodge, "A Visit to Queen Alexandra Solarium," pp. 242-243; E. Frances Upton, "Tuberculosis Nursing in Sanitoria," pp. 243-246.

[27] Elizabeth Smellie, "The Nurse and Her Opportunities," CN, Vol. XXIV, No.10, October 1928, pp. 520-523.

[28] Elizabeth L. Smellie, "Rural Nursing," ICN, July 12, 1929, and Alexandra M. Walker, "Rural Nursing," ICN, July 11, 1929, OCHA.

[29] A Student Nurse, "Progress and Opportunities in the Field of Nursing," CN, Vol. XXV, No.3, March 1929, p. 131.

[30] "The Private Duty Nurse and the Association," CN, Vol. XXIV, No.2, February 1923, p. 101 and Annie E. McIntyre, "Nursing as a Profession," CN, Vol. XXVI, No.10, October 1925, p. 526.

[31] Myrtle E. Kay, "The Private Duty Nurse," CN, Vol. XXVII, No.4, April 1926, p. 192.

[32] "Miss Sarah Edith Young," CN, Vol. XXIV, No.7, July 1928, p. 14.

[33] "Essays on Nursing Ethics," CN, Vol. XIX, No.5, May 1923, pp. 288-291.

[34] Florence H. Walker, "Why Be a Nurse," CN, vol. XIX, No.7, July 1923, p. 408.

[35] W. Gordon M. Byers M.D., "The Ideals of Nursing," CN. Vol. XVIII, No.2, February 1922, p. 90.

[36] Isabel Irvine, "Nursing on the Prairies," unpublished paper, ND, p.4, OCHA.

[37] Edith Young, "Insights of 54 Years of Nursing Experience in Thirty Minutes," ND, p.4, Author's Possession. Young went on to become the Director of Nursing at the Ottawa Civic Hospital and retired from that position during the sixties.

[38] Sybil Brower, Videotaped interview, Vulcan, Alberta, 1988 and Edith Henry, Audiotaped interview, Calgary, Alberta, 1994.

[39] Ethel Johns, "The Challenge of the Future," CN, Vol. XXVII, No.1, January 1921, pp. 5-10 and "Letters to the Editor," CN, Vol. XVII, No.3, March 1921, pp. 156-160.

[40] A. Gaskell, "Report Private Duty Nursing Section Committee," CN, Vol. XVII, No.7, July 1921, p. 453.

[41] Edith Gaskell, "Private Duty Nursing Department," CN, Vol. XVII, No.11, November 1921, p. 690.

[42] Helen Carruthers, "Private Duty Nursing," CN, Vol. XXIII, No.9, September 1927, p. 479.

[43] "Canadian Nurses Association Minutes - General Meetings," 1924, MG28-I248, M4605, NAC.

[44] I.H. Cameron. "The Nurses Life and Calling," Toronto, 1922, p. 6, 7. Paper presented to CNATN, OCHA.

[45] Heather MacDougall, Activists and Advocates, pp. 65,66.

[46] Elizabeth Smellie, "The Nurse and Her Opportunities," CN, Vol. XXIV, No.10, October 1928, p. 523.

[47] Quoted in Gibbon and Mathewson, Three Centuries, p. 371.

[48] "Alberta Association for Graduate Nurses Official Minutes," Vol. 1, p.151, AARNA.

[49] "Resolutions Passed at the General Meeting," 1924, p. 30, CNA Minutes 1924-1932, MG28-I-248, Reel M-4605,NAC.

[50] "AAGN Official Minutes," Vol.1, pp. 177-179, AARNA.

[51] Eunice Dyke, "Report of the Annual Meeting of the National Council of Women, 1927," CN, Vol. XXIV, No.7, July 1928, pp. 15,16. Perhaps the brevity of midwifery training programs was one reason for the opposition among nursing leaders.

[52] Leslie Bell, "Nurses and their Attitude Towards Sex," CN, Vol. XXIV, No.10, October 1928, p. 525.

[53] Elizabeth W. Odell, "Eliminating the Unfit from the School of Nursing," CN, Vol. XXV, No.12, December 1929, pp. 723-724.

[54] E. W. McKinnon, "Wide-Awake," CN, Vol. XXI, No.5, May 1925, pp. 247-248.

[55] Adelaide M. Plumptre, "Caught Napping," CN, Vol. XXI, No.1, January 1925, pp. 5-8 and J.P. Page, "Medical Aspects of Immigration," CN, Vol. XXV, No.8, August 1929, pp. 395-399.

[56] E. Stanley Ryerson M.D., C.M. "The Preparation of a Curriculum," presented July 9, 1929 at ICN Meeting in Montreal, p. 2. OCHA.

[57] Ibid., p. 3, 8.

[58] Michael Sadler, "Brains in Nursing," CN, Vol. XIX, No.6, June 1923, pp. 327,330.

[59] Dr. Dunlop, "Address," CN, Vol. XXI, No.7, July 1925, p. 363.

[60] "Psychology and Nursing," CLP, December, 1927, pp. 163-164 and "The Study of Nursing Conditions," CLP, February, 1930, pp. 46-48.

[61] M.J. Marsh, "Reasons Why Some Nurses Fail," TNHR, June, 1920, pp. 573-574.

[62] L.J. Carter, "Some Present-Day Problems of the Nursing Profession," CN, Vol. XVII, No.3, March 1921, p. 150.

[63] W. Gordon Byers, "The Ideals of Nursing," CN, Vol. XVIII, No.2, February 1922, pp. 85-90 and Irving Cameron, "The Nurse's Life and Calling," CN, Vol. XVIII, No.10, October 1922, pp. 636-642.

[64] Henry M.W. Gray, "Nurses' Graduating Exercises," CLP, August, 1929, pp. 47-51.

[65] "Sarah Edith Young," CN, Vol. XXIV, No.7, July 1928, p. 14.

[66] Stewart Cameron, "Nursing Problems," CN, Vol. XXIII, No.10, October 1927, pp. 520-527.

[67] John M. Gunn, "Nurses - Here and There: A Few Glimpses and Some Reflections," CN, Vol. XXIV, No.7, July 1928, p. 347.

[68] Gladys Moon Jones, "Women of the A.E.F.," LHJ, November, 1928-May, 1929.

[69] "Part of an Address Before the Hamilton Health Association," January 19, 1920, author unknown, B72-0005-005, UTA.

[70] Ida F. Butler, "How to Nurse the Nursing Profession," LHJ, April, 1921, p.12.

[71] Margaret S. McWilliams, "A Laywoman's View of the Private Duty Nurse," CN, Vol. XVII, No.1, January 1921, p. 20.

[72] "As Seen By A Patient," CN, Vol. XVIII, No.2, February 1922, p. 70.

[73] "'Oh Wad the Power The Giftie Gie Us To See Oursels as Ithers See Us': A Symposium on Nurses By Patients," TNHR, Vol 79, No.2, August 1927, pp. 147-150.

[74] LHJ, December, 1925, p.1; October, 1926, p. 132; January, 1927, p. 44; June, 1930, p. 87; February, 1931, pp. 68,69; March, 1931, p. 161; February, 1933, p. 100; April, 1934, p. 117; July, 1934, p. 97; October, 1934, p. 137; December, 1934, p. 54; September, 1937, pp. 44,82; January, 1938, p. 54; May, 1938, p. 123.

[75] "Toronto General," March, 1920, author unknown, B-27-005-003, UTA.

Chapter Four

WEATHERING THE ECONOMIC STORM: THE 1930S

On May 6, 1933, <u>The Toronto Daily Star</u> reported on a reception held for Miss Eunice Dyke, former supervisor of public health nursing in Toronto, at which she was:

> hailed as a pioneer in the field of public health nursing and as one of the first to give proper recognition to the value of preventive medicine. She was eulogized as a "faithful public servant" and tribute was paid to her 21 years spent in assisting to build up the health department to a point where it attained world-wide recognition.[1]

This was not a "post-funeral" reception but a gathering held to acknowledge the contributions made by Eunice Dyke during her career in the Toronto Department of Public Health. Eunice Dyke, for all intents and purposes, had been fired by the Medical Officer of Health in 1932. His decision, upheld by the Toronto City Council, effectively ended her nursing career. The incident that sparked the conflict is complicated but involved Eunice Dyke challenging the dismissal of one of her nursing staff; in doing so, she posed a threat to the Medical Officer of Health. The entire drama was aired in the media. Eunice Dyke survived this humiliation and later became a social activist for seniors. Her experiences bear considerable similarity to the situation encountered by Canadian nurses in general during the thirties, experiences that they survived as well.

The Thirties was a decade in which nursing faced stiff opposition on the road to professionalism: resistance to improved educational qualifications and preparation, unemployment, difficult conditions of work, and occasional wholesale opposition to its very existence. Canadians in general were in a mood of apprehension, which included discontent with traditionally accepted Canadian institutions, one of which was nursing service. Still, the publication of <u>The Survey of Nursing Education in Canada</u>, or better known as the "Weir Report" in 1932, provided nursing with solid ammunition to support its professional vision. This report not only validated the nursing leadership's desire for improved and advanced education for nurses but also recommended that government funds be directed to support such advances.

Nurses appeared to be divided when faced with the need to identify a solution that would assist them in "weathering the storm." Although tension within nursing persisted, all three nursing groups were working separately to create a permanent niche for nursing within health care and in so doing contributed to paving the road to professionalism. Nursing leaders continued to follow through on strategies that would shift nursing from the status of spiritual vocation to that of a secular profession. Of prime importance for nursing educators in particular was the environment in which education took place. They focused their attention on the need to move general nursing education from the hospital to the university and to standardize nursing education. Success in this venture was a direct result of the effort and commitment of individual nurses. Private duty nurses focused on the importance of surviving the deprivation caused by the unemployment of the 1930s. The strategies employed by this group of nurses brought nursing to a higher level of indispensability in Canadian health care and, as such, supported the professional goals of nursing leaders. Public health nurses continued to work towards bringing their work into the realm of accepted public service. Consequently, the public health nurse continued to move nursing service outside of the hospital into the broader community and establish an independent nursing presence that interacted with everyone, not just the sick. This would also further professional goals. The efforts of these three groups to "weather the storm" culminated in a unified movement to shift nursing from vocation to profession. Survival is the key to understanding this situation and the fact that nurses not only survived but made significant steps in the accomplishment of this undertaking is related to their integration into Canadian society in general.

The Canadian climate appeared to be somewhat receptive to these tactics. Nevertheless, all three nursing groups encountered opposition from the medical profession. During the 1930s, nursing and medicine appeared to be moving on a collision path, particularly regarding the territorial concerns of public health. The economic downturn drew physicians together in their shared grievances because of the unprecedented decline in their incomes. They mobilized politically and mounted strong campaigns for medical relief payments. Physicians incorporated a variety of strategies and most supported the opinion that some form of state-aided health insurance was inevitable. In support of this belief, the Canadian Medical Association made its case to the federal government based on the premise that the medical profession's first duty was the protection of the public health. Physicians and politicians alike accepted the fact that physicians, nurses, and hospitals would be competing for payment from the health insurance fund, as opposed to that of the patient.[2] This emerging competitive relationship created inevitable opportunities for confrontation as nursing strove for professional status. These confrontations then contributed to a fluctuation in public support that revealed itself in the confused popular image of the nurse, an image that vacillated between good and evil.

Any success realized by the profession was due, in part, to the fact that Canadians were occupied with many other issues. The economic reality of the "dirty thirties" resulted in dramatic ideological shifts for many Canadians. Ideologies such as pacifism, socialism, and spiritual revivalism became popular and were later rejected. Divisions that emerged regionally, ethnically, and along class lines brought with them the voice of dissent. Not surprisingly, much political alienation was voiced across the country as well.[3] Taken together, it is clear that the disturbances apparent in the economic, social and intellectual climate reflected a society in turmoil – one that had much to occupy itself. Therefore, the nursing situation was left to those who possessed a vested interest.

No Canadian survived the 1930s without some scars but the two groups most affected were the unemployed and the prairie farmer. The problems of the Depression were not easily solved and the experience of those years demanded that Canadians seriously begin to analyze the structure of their society and the role of social institutions. Further, they questioned the accepted values in political and economic life, and debated radical ideas that only a few years earlier would have been ridiculed as utopian or heretical. The Depression forced Canadians to turn inwards in order to discover the solution to their economic problems. Society looked to the federal government for the expertise that would repair the damage that had occurred. In this respect, the decade was one of centralization, one that transferred much of the fiscal and intellectual stresses from the provinces to Ottawa. Out of this expansion in federal government activity emerged the beginnings of Canada as a welfare state. This was accompanied by the emergence of government experts, or the men who would later become key administrators in the implementation of new social policies.[4]

Intellectual expertise was in demand and thrived during the 1930s. This resulted in the formation of an intellectual elite based in the universities of the country. This elite developed connections with the politicians through their strong desire to assume their proper role as leaders of society in a time of crisis. They held the general view that "efficiency must serve the

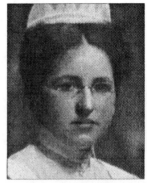

LEFT: Eunice Dyck, a public health nurse in Toronto who became famous for tackling the Medical Officer of Health in support of her nurses.

BOTTOM: Ann Hammill, Birth Control Nurse, with a client family in Alberta. (Courtesy University of Toronto Archives)

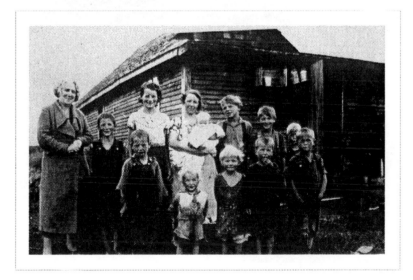

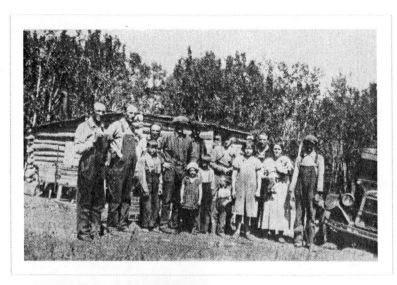

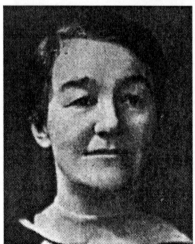

TOP: Typical prairie family which might be visited by the Birth Control nurse.

BOTTOM: Marion Lindeburgh, Director of the School of Nursing at McGill University during the establishment of the degree nursing program. Nurses from across Canada contributed to the funding of the program. (Courtesy Helen K. Mussallem Library)

common weal, and ... if the humanitarian task is honestly performed, we will have the basis of an enduring efficiency."[5] This notion suggests that it would be possible to meet the needs of society through programs that combined humanitarianism and efficiency. The experts who would inspire this systematic planning process were the social scientists and the implementing agent would be the state.

Nurses too, were influenced by the plethora of ideas surfacing during the thirties, but their plans were sometimes restricted by their gender. It is true that by 1930, societal attitudes were changing and that many liberal thinkers gave their enthusiastic support to women who wished to pursue non-traditional professions. But conservative attitudes continued to prevail in institutions such as the university. For example, as more and more women joined the teaching profession, one university professor commented, "no university teacher wants to be condemned to teaching women. He knows that that means an old age of pedantry, or empty, meaningless aestheticism."[6] In the face of this gender bias, ambitious, successful women often faced opposition in the society of the thirties. When they sought respect for that in which they had invested so much of themselves, they were usually rewarded only by other professional women. There was a distinct need for working women to support each other. Margaret McWilliams, a contemporary feminist who operated from a privileged position, noted "women needed to retain and develop women's sense of solidarity in order to achieve equality."[7] Therefore, to make any progress, nurses would have to maintain some sense of unity and they managed to do this within their separate clinical groupings.

The inclination of society to look for solutions in intellectual expertise supported nursing's professional aspirations. Consequently, nursing leaders continued to work towards the improvement of nursing education and were convinced that the ideal setting for this education was within the university environment. Indeed, the <u>Survey of Nursing Education in</u>

Canada, published in 1932, acknowledged "nursing should be regarded as a profession, however immature in the attainment of professional standards, rather than as a potential member of a trade union." Given the reduced economic resources of the time, this statement was probably motivated by the need to discourage demands for higher pay. Nursing leaders, however, saw it as a means to attain their vision for nursing and nursing education.

The Canadian Nurses Association financed seventy percent of the cost of the Survey and the Canadian Medical Association the remaining thirty. As Dr. G.Stewart Cameron noted in the "Foreword":

> As hospitals increased by the score a multiplicity of opinions arose not only on the academic training of students, but on the whole problem of the nurse in her relationship to the hospital, the medical profession and the public at large.[8]

The committee examined all areas of nursing and published a detailed, lengthy, and comprehensive report. Although this report was important for nursing education and nursing's legitimacy at the time, it was also significant in that it was the first occasion on which an "outsider" participated in an investigation of nursing and furthermore, was allowed to make recommendations.

The Survey attracted a good deal of attention from various sectors of Canadian society. Weir suggested that schools of nursing be incorporated into the general educational system of the country and be subsidized by government funds. Given the timing, the Canadian economic climate was such that to place more stress on the taxpayer would necessarily attract attention. However, Weir viewed the nurse as indispensable and thus gave justification for his conclusion:

> who else than the trained nurse can possibly be in the strategic position to act as liaison officer between the 'values and virtues' of the old and rapidly passing school of medicine and the scientific efficiency of the new? No one but

the nurse is in the field for this supreme venture. If she fails, the case is lost by default. Nor can she succeed unless she be competent to carry out in the sickroom the instructions of the modern specialist in the spirit with the humanitarian touch of the erstwhile medical generalist. Unless she be a woman of superior capacity, thoroughly educated in her art, there can be little likelihood either that the best of the old will be maintained or that the best of the new be added.[9]

The editor of The Canadian Nurse noted at the time that Weir had shifted from his normally neutral position "to one of keen and understanding sympathy towards nursing" during the collection of the data for the report.[10]

The Canadian Nurses Association took the findings of the Survey and immediately developed a list of recommendations to be sent to all of the provincial associations for action. The main recommendation was to move towards higher and more uniform educational standards. "Joint Study Committees" were established at the provincial level and by 1933, three provinces had considered and adopted many of the recommendations of the Canadian Nurses Association.[11] This would suggest a fair degree of unity and support for these ideas both nationally and locally. Public support was reflected in The Honourable Vincent Massey's presentation to the Canadian Nurses Association entitled, "The Public and the Survey" and in an article by Reba Riddell, published in The Canadian Forum entitled, "Nurses and Nursing."[12]

The Survey concluded that since student nurses were dealing with human values and needs, with human problems and outlooks as were teachers, lawyers and doctors, that the solution to the problems of nursing education was to be found in the university. The committee agreed that:

A university setting and status, apart from the provision of superior facilities for investigation and research, will probably give the study of nursing problems a true dignity and attract a better average type of student ... The field of nursing is bristling with problems that challenge solution and herein is offered a great opportunity for Canadian universities to render a real public service.[13]

In this way, Weir gave leaders in nursing education the encouragement they needed to continue their efforts in the cause of improved nursing education, efforts that would promote professionalism as well.

Kathleen Russell at the University of Toronto undertook one local initiative. Russell was Director of the Department of Public Health Nursing in which the University offered a one-year certificate course that prepared graduate nurses for work in public health. She was also working toward the establishment of a school of nursing within the university that would function independently and free from hospital control. Tenacious and determined, Russell achieved success in 1932 when the School of Nursing at the University of Toronto was awarded funding by both the Ontario government and the Rockefeller Foundation.[14] In 1933, the School opened its doors "to remain financially independent of all hospitals, while having access to their patients for clinical teaching and accepting complete responsibility for the students."[15] The importance of this step lies in the removal of nursing education from the control of the hospitals where the labour of the student nurses had been exploited. Russell's program was not a degree program simply because she wanted the preparation of nurses in the new School to attain university standards before launching a Baccalaureate program. This decision was in accordance with a recommendation of The Survey that stated that "until such nursing courses are well established and of undoubtedly high standards, diplomas, instead of degrees, should be awarded."[16]

Throughout these developments at Toronto, Russell worked under the watchful eye of the Medical Faculty. Initial approval from Medicine was required before she could even set her plan in motion.[17] In order to ensure the participation of Medicine in the development of the School, it was recommended that five members of the Medical Faculty be involved with the School of Nursing. Between 1934 and 1939, physicians outnumbered nurses on most of the committees, and most notably on the Executive Committee that, in 1939, had six physicians and only three nurses. The membership of the Examinations Committee and the Curriculum Committee fluctuated back and forth and the Applications Committee usually numbered more nurses than physicians.[18] This was one example of the continued interest the medical profession had in nursing education, perhaps out of fear of losing control of it. By 1936, the School continued to operate independently, and Russell gave a cautious but optimistic report in The Canadian Nurse.

Marion Lindeburgh paralleled Kathleen Russell's tireless efforts at Toronto at McGill University. In 1932, the university administration recommended the closure of the Nursing School because the university was not prepared to offer any financial support. Nurses from across Canada donated $30,000.00 to keep the school open. In 1938, as a result of this financial support, the Board of Governors gave definite assurance that the school had the full support of the University and the personal interest of the Governors. Practical evidence of this interest and support was shown in the administration's decision to aid the School in balancing its budget during the next five years.[19]

Lindeburgh's program was only a Diploma Program but her efforts and success were completely dependent on the support she received from Canadian nurses. For example, the Ottawa Civic Hospital nursing students had a small amount deducted from their already small stipend without giving their consent for the deduction. Lindeburgh was fully aware of the possibility of a change of heart among the Board of Governors and announced that the Alumnae Association would be "going forward with plans for raising a permanent endowment fund" for the newly-named "School of Nursing, McGill University."[20] In this university as well, the continued existence of nursing studies was questionable, at best.

The shift of nursing education from the hospital to the independent setting of the university represented an attempt on the part of nurse educators to incorporate science into the art of nursing education. In 1936, these efforts were further supported by the publication of A Proposed Curriculum for Schools of Nursing in Canada. This Curriculum was the work of a national curriculum committee, formed in 1932 and chaired by Marion Lindeburgh. The adoption of the Curriculum would not only standardize nursing education but also encourage the goal that nurses "be able at all times to invite confidence, to manifest a real interest in human problems and to render the kind of assistance which typifies the spirit and practice of an indispensable professional service."[21] Therefore, the efforts of the national organization were in harmony with the vision of professionalism that motivated local initiatives.

The Canadian Nurses Association continually worked "toward the provision of a better nursing service for Canada and improved conditions for nurses from the educational, legislative, social, and economic standpoints."[22] These efforts necessitated their involvement with other organizations whose work overlapped that of nursing. In particular, the Canadian Nurses Association directed considerable effort into equalizing its relationship with the Canadian Hospital Council and the Canadian Medical Association. George Weir, along with physicians and representatives from the Rockefeller Foundation were invited to attend the 1936 biennial meeting in Vancouver. Their enthusiastic response encouraged the association to invite the Canadian Hospital Council and the Canadian Medical Association to the biennial meeting in 1938. At the 1938 meeting, Ruby Simpson, the President of the Canadian Nurses Association, expressed her wish to continue to work towards their goals. These were:

Professional unity and understanding through self-criticism and appraisal; the development of our <u>Journal</u> as a continued means of communication; a growing, changing educational programme; willingness to make a real effort to improve our service to the community; a desire to stand with other countries in contributing to world progress in nursing.[23]

In spite of the inclusion of members of the medical profession at these meetings, nurses received mixed messages from them. One physician made a plea for moderation in nursing education because he felt that there was a limit to the financial burden that could be borne by the public and those hospitals owned by the public.[24] At the same time, Dr. Attlee, a Halifax physician who regularly contributed to <u>The Canadian Nurse</u>, urged nurses to make for themselves within medicine the same sort of world that architects have made within Engineering.[25] This physician appeared to support nursing as a secular profession. Nursing leaders were resolute in pursuing this goal and, to this end, involved themselves in Canadian politics.

The economic hardships of the Thirties, coupled with federal-provincial jurisdictional confusion, demanded the attention of the politicians. In 1937, the government appointed a Royal Commission to investigate Dominion-Provincial Relations. The Commission members were drawn from the intellectual elite and provided a vehicle by which the public and the provinces could be brought to the same position as the intellectual community. The expectation of the report was that it would be a mature statement of the creed of modern social and economic planning. According to historian Doug Owram, the Commission was an expression of a particular set of problems facing Canada as well as a reflection of the mind-set of the intellectual community by the late 1930s. Therefore, it mirrored a particular group of intellectual, social, and economic reformers who, so its members argued, sought to preserve the original vision of Confederation.[26]

113

The Canadian Nurses Association also participated in this commission. Their "Submission to the Royal Commission on Dominion-Provincial Relations" portrayed the Canadian Nurses Association as a national association committed to creating unity and mutual understanding among the provincial associations. The Canadian Nurses Association was also committed to the provision of quality nursing service to Canadians, and recommended that the organized nursing profession be afforded an opportunity of serving in an advisory capacity on any committee created to investigate, establish and oversee such a plan.[27] Canadian nurses, therefore, participated in concerns affecting mainstream Canadian society and reflected their willingness to become involved.

Nevertheless, nursing continued to encounter opposition from many members of the medical profession. Physicians denied the fact that student nurses were exploited for service to the hospital. They also expressed concern that the profession was becoming overcrowded due to the over-production of ill-prepared nurses. This situation was quickly linked to the economic crisis. Although the Survey recommended an improved and standardized educational preparation for nurses, the medical profession feared that this would result in over trained and expensive nurses:

> Of all the dangerous symptoms ... confronting the medical profession and the national economics, there is none more menacing than the overtrained, superlatively expensive nurse, who is perhaps the most salient and untoward feature in the approaching crisis of over-standardization in the care of the sick.[28]

Physicians next expressed concern about the unnecessary teaching of theory in the education of nurses and the lessening emphasis on the practical because in their opinion, "the duty of the nurse ... is still that of making the patient comfortable. The care of the patient is nursing. The cure of the patient is mainly the practice of medicine."[29] Clearly, for this physician, little theory was required for the maintenance of the comfort of the patient. Furthermore, to improve nursing educational programs, nursing had only to turn to the medical profession to assist in the creation of the best system for the education and training of the nurse.[30]

The recommendations that resulted from the Survey provided encouragement for the nursing leaders to actively pursue their vision. For nursing leaders, the solution to the problems confronting nurses was to be found in an improved and standardized educational preparation. To this end, any opposition proffered by the medical profession only gave nurses the incentive to pursue their goal with more tenacity and determination.

The experience of the private duty nurse was considerably different. They weathered the harsh realities by adapting their nursing service to the changing economic climate. The perception that there did indeed exist an oversupply of nurses was a direct result of the unemployment that was the experience of most nurses. Nurses, however, met the hardships of the Depression by drawing together and supporting each other. For example, nursing service was often given in exchange for room and board in the hospital rather than wages.[31] Acquiescence to this strategy was motivated primarily by the desire on the part of the nurse to deliver quality nursing care to the sick and to feed herself. Adaptation and survival was the motivating factor behind all of the actions of the graduate nurses. Moreover, in spite of the difficulties encountered in the experience of the private duty nurse, her response established nursing service as an indispensable asset to the community. As well, local initiatives to improve working conditions enhanced nursing as an acceptable career choice. This line of action contributed to the leadership's vision of professionalism in that it maintained nursing as an active and viable force in health care.

The predicament of the graduate nurses during the thirties appeared to be insurmountable. Their growing numbers among the unemployed supported the perception that there existed an oversupply. This situation was simply a product of the depressed circumstances of the day. Indeed, as the thirties progressed the situation deteriorated, thus demanding innovative strategies. It was noted in 1933, "that nurses and actresses show more adaptability in finding occupation than any other woman[sic]."[32] Nurses themselves recommended adaptability to their private duty-nursing colleagues seeking employment. One suggestion made by another private duty nurse, was to develop special accomplishments:

> If you nurse children, practice telling children's stories until you do it well ... learn something of occupational therapy. Children love to work with their hands. For obstetrical cases learn short cuts in baby care; know about time schedules; study best authorities on supplementary diets. If you are nursing men, learn Bridge and card games that two can play; watch stock quotations and discuss them.[33]

In spite of the adjustments made to the changing situation, the private duty nurse was criticized on many levels and this led to tense and confused interactions with national leaders and with the Canadian public. The fact that the nurse expected a fee for her services exposed her to criticism. She was accused of being commercial and of lacking that real feeling of service normally associated with a 'true nurse'. The professional and financial hardships experienced by graduate nurses during the thirties led to the following observation:

> Nurses, as a group, on this continent are not happy looking: they are ... much more frequently bored and cynical looking ... the public is not dissatisfied with modern nursing technique which is assuredly much more efficient than ever before. Nevertheless, the public is not entirely satisfied with nurses.[34]

Nurses had every reason to be unhappy. The public wanted their services but was unwilling to provide sufficient financial remuneration for those services. Nurses had difficulty organizing themselves to fight the apparent condition of imbalance that brought prolonged hardship and unnecessary suffering to this large branch of nursing and to a great many sick people in the community.[35] The private duty group, in particular, felt isolated from the other groups in nursing. An example of this was noted when an opinion survey of the various levels of nursing was taken in 1939, regarding the idea that nurses were "emancipated." All of the nurses agreed that nurses were emancipated except for one private duty nurse who remarked:

> I haven't noticed anything different. I still don't know that there's a definite connection between speaking up about things and getting work. If you have too many opinions you can't get work to do. So I keep still as well as I ever did.[36]

The despondency apparent in the tone of this nurse's words reflects the dependency for employment that nurses had on the good will of the physician. This condition of work would only add to their frustration. However, the majority of these nurses continued with the struggle to maintain nursing as a worthwhile career for women to pursue. Efforts to ensure the survival of nursing would clearly further the professional vision. In order to do this, they turned their attention to working conditions and the working environment.

Discussions about working conditions addressed questions of salary, lack of pensions, and the lengthy hours of work. Many narratives, such as the following, were published regarding the actual work situation:

> I found I was to be on duty twenty-four hours and sleep on a cot in the patient's room, and wash and dress in an adjoining room. Everyone visiting the patient came through this room. One day I had a narrow escape as the minister came through without knocking just as I finished dressing.[37]

In spite of these and other multiple hardships endured by some private duty nurses, compensation was seldom monetary but offered in terms of the kindness and appreciation of the patients and their families. The national association discussed the problem of excessive hours of work for private duty nurses employed in the hospital. However, it was at the local level that concrete modifications materialized.

Nurses in London, Ontario were supported by the hospital administration, the physicians, and the community, in their initiatives towards the incorporation of eight-hour duty on March 1, 1934. Their purpose was three-fold:

1. More work for nurses
2. More even distribution of work
3. Extra service to the public.[38]

Previously, two twelve hour shifts cost $10.00 at $5.00 per shift but the eight hour shift would only cost $3.00 therefore, a patient would receive twenty-four hours of nursing care for a dollar less at $9.00. This announcement was made with great optimism but it was noted in <u>The Canada Lancet and Practitioner</u> a few months later, that it was highly unlikely that any level of government in Canada would furnish the necessary funds to support health insurance or shortened hours of work for nurses.[39]

The eight-hour day also became the subject of much discussion among nurses. As one nurse asked:

Is there any other profession, or other branch of the nursing profession in which one must needs spend from twelve to twenty hours a day with patients (or people) in their weakest, most miserable, most critical condition, and yet be cheerful under both praise and abuse, realizing that the sick are not responsible, and that their friends are overtaxed with anxiety?[40]

To alleviate the obvious problems associated with the long hours of duty, the eight-hour day was related to the benefits that would be enjoyed by the patient, the physician, the hospital, and even for the greater good of the public.[41] The notion, however, was controversial and sparked considerable debate. Physicians thought the addition of another nurse would disturb the patient. For this group, the solution to the problem of unemployed nurses was not the eight-hour day but a reduction in the fee charged to the patient. There was also the problem of the more senior nurses being unwilling to work a shorter shift because it represented a reduction in their income. It was noted that this would oblige them to drop the insurance they had been carrying to provide them with post-retirement security.[42]

Nonetheless, success was achieved in some provinces at the local level and reported enthusiastically in The Canadian Nurse. The medical profession delivered the strongest opposition but the general public accepted these shortened hours with "surprisingly little difficulty." It was noted that this was more difficult to do in private homes but modification of the twelve-hour day was possible.[43] In spite of these local initiatives, most Canadian nurses continued to work under trying and exhausting conditions.

Conditions were so deplorable for one nurse that after fourteen years in the profession, she concluded that she had "The Right to Live" and withdrew from nursing. This particular nurse had grown tired of the fact that:

> The nursing day still started at 7 A.M. and still ended at 7:30 P.M. and often later. My off-duty time during this period, unless spent in complete rest, meant that one was unfit to carry on efficiently after returning to duty; so broadly speaking (except for meal-times), one gave that whole eleven hours to duty daily. Such a working situation carried on day after day and week after week, seems to me ... incompatible with the high standards of nursing service which good nursing requires.[44]

Most nurses, however, remained loyal to their work and investigated other strategies of protest. This was the case for a small number of nurses in Comox, British Columbia who chose strike action.

The situation at St. Joseph's Hospital shared many similarities with the above anecdote. In addition, the nurses were required to "*live in*," they had little time off, and there was no overtime pay, holiday pay, or sick pay. Out of their $90.00 monthly wage, the nurses paid $30.00 for room and board and were responsible for their own laundry costs. The nurses, frustrated with the hospital management's refusal to improve the work situation, walked off the job on April 12, 1939 and returned on April 18, 1939 with the promise of improved working conditions. These nurses received support from their community, the Chief of Staff, and the local Member of Parliament. But they received only disapproval from their provincial association because according to historian Jo Ann Whittaker:

> It was more important, in 1939, to maintain the professional image than to agitate for improved working conditions. Nurses did not become involved in controversial issues.[45]

Strike activity seemed to represent a direct refutation of professionalism as well as contrary to the older idea of nursing as a vocation that continued to be the issue at the forefront of nursing discussions.

Other local initiatives in response to the unemployment situation were not publicized and support by the professional organization was not always forthcoming. The Calgary Group Nursing Society, formed in 1934, undertook one such initiative. This group organized under a Board of Directors that consisted of seven nurses and had an Advisory Committee made up of four laymen and three professional men (a dentist, a lawyer and a physician). The group offered nursing service at a minimum cost on an insurance basis and employed thirty qualified nurses.[46] In the beginning, both the provincial and the national associations applauded the group's efforts, but in 1935, when the Group launched a sweepstake and sold tickets that provided one hour of nursing service a curtain of disapproval was lowered. Such action was considered unprofessional and contrary to the aims and objectives of the Canadian Nurses Association. In spite of the lack of support from the Association, the Group succeeded for four years only to disappear in 1938.[47]

The Alberta Association of Registered Nurses did support and, indeed, conducted and financed "An Educational Experiment" at Alder Flats, Alberta. The goal was to provide nursing service to a rural community where it was needed. A supplemental goal was to train an unemployed graduate nurse in district nursing. Clearly, this represented a pulling together of the nursing community to assist in the survival of one of its members.[48]

Another Alberta example of mutual support among nurses was the creation of a Mutual Benefit and Loan Fund from which unemployed graduate nurses could draw when they were faced with serious financial embarrassment. One writer noted that "the appeal for funds was met with a very generous response and a substantial sum was collected."[49] Given the nature of the desperate economic times, it should not be surprising that nurses were concerned with their practice and their survival. Nursing practice took up most of the attention of the graduate nurse.

One enterprising nurse in Nova Scotia directed her attention to the need of frail infants for an incubator. Due to the lack of funds, the hospital administration could not approve any expenditure for such an item. Not to be discouraged, "Miss Boa ingeniously improvised and had an inexpensive but efficient incubator made out of an ordinary wash boiler at a total of $8.50."[50] Ingenuity was the norm for nurses during the Depression years and recognition of the need for this kept all of their attention focused on the task at hand.

Up until 1936, Isabel Irvine, a nurse practicing in rural Saskatchewan, delivered thirty babies without the assistance of an anesthetic or a physician. One delivery required all of her skills and deserves a full account:

> My only breech delivery was the worst. It was in the middle of the winter and the husband had to travel seven or eight miles with horses and a big sleigh. There was no phone so he was unable to forewarn me of his arrival ... By the time we arrived at the home of the pregnant woman, the horses were over-heated and the husband had to put them in the barn immediately. I went to the house myself and found the wife, who couldn't speak English. She was walking around with the baby's feet hanging down from her. I had to get her to understand that she had to get onto the bed so that I could deliver the baby. I was sure it's little neck would be broken. However, I got her on the bed and, knowing there wasn't much time, I took the two ankles between my fingers and swung the baby over backwards. I put the finger of my other hand in it's mouth and was ready to pull with the next pain. It was a girl. By the time I had cleaned up the baby, mother and myself, the baby seemed alright.[51]

Dramatic situations such as these offered nurses valuable opportunities to prove their usefulness to society while their skills and dedication enhanced the value of nursing service.

Similarly, nurses practicing in rural hospitals contributed to the growing importance of nursing. The nurse was often required to fulfill the roles of cook, laundress, anesthetist, surgical assistant and even janitor. As Edith Young, later Director of Nursing at the Ottawa Civic Hospital, recalled:

> The janitor imbibed a bit too much at times and I recall the night that my assistant and I climbed a ladder to the loft of a barn belonging to the hospital and with ice tongs, secured ice which was required for a tonsil clinic the next day, when specialists in ear, nose and throat came from Ottawa. The usual time for MAJOR operations was between 1 AM and 4

AM when trains were available for surgeons to come to Almonte and return to Ottawa.[52]

This experience was not unusual. It was true for graduate nurses across Canada.

Nursing practice, nursing service, science and professionalism became part of the rhetoric associated with the rank-and-file nurses. For some, professional nursing was linked to the phenomenal developments occurring in science that necessitated an improved nursing education. In order to create pride and commitment to the profession, nurses were reminded, "the health of a nation depends on its women."[53] Even the selection of students was based on professional motive and attitude, or a "high call to service and sincerity."[54] The Canadian Nurse published letters from graduate nurses praising the service component of professional nursing. These nurses expressed concern in these letters that some nurses might have lost their way in that they regarded nursing as a livelihood and not as a dedication to the relief of the sick and suffering.[55] The earlier ideal of nursing as a vocation coincided with the new ideal of nursing as a profession at this point. What was once religious virtue became secular virtue. Vestiges of the earlier ideal remained, however, especially among private duty nurses. The need for unselfishness and self-sacrifice was further underlined in a questionnaire published in "The Private Duty Section" of The Canadian Nurse, in 1938, entitled "Are You a Good Nurse?." According to this questionnaire, if one was a good nurse, one answered twenty-four of the twenty-eight questions correctly. That is to say that one was fit, literate, unselfish, humble, happy at all times and in possession of a certain amount of religious awe.[56]

For the typical graduate nurse the decade opened with admonitions to keep nursing alive. When there was some concern that nursing was drifting, organizational concerns rose to the surface of the discussion as in the following:

> Could not a strong body representing modern nursing be formed, prepared to take strong and vigorous action to save the wreckage, and see what can be done to reconstruct the whole nursing profession.[57]

To this end, the national organization encouraged all nurses to contribute their time and talent to their provincial association in order to ensure that the aims of the nursing profession would be realized. Indeed, this support was often associated with romantic notions of duty:

> No one can live to himself, and just as you have a duty to your fellow men, you have a duty to your own kind. Be loyal to your profession, by supporting the efforts of its representatives; do your share in reaching the goal when all the sick shall be cared for and all the nurses occupied therewith.[58]

Although the tone of this summons is similar to a nineteenth-century appeal from Nightingale, the focus had changed. Nurses now expressed loyalty to professional ideas that would ensure the survival of nursing after the Depression. The outbreak of war in 1939 gave nursing further assurance of its survival when nurses directed all of their attention and effort to military service. Once again, as in World War I, Canadian nurses were reminded by their national organization to be steadfast, courageous and devoted in their willingness to serve.[59]

Grass roots nursing not only survived the thirties but also managed to maintain a certain amount of independence in spite of the dim view of this position taken by the medical profession. Physicians considered the nursing profession to be an auxiliary to the medical profession therefore; physicians were to be sympathetic and helpful to the "junior profession."[60] Indeed, if allowed, the senior profession would assist the junior profession to cure itself. Moreover, all problems would be solved if the nursing profession would only produce nurses who conformed to the ideal envisioned by the medical profession.

One example of this ideal was Mary Agnes Snively, Superintendent of Nurses at the Toronto General Hospital, whose memory Canadian physicians resurrected in 1934. They described her to be a "Canadian Nightingale" because:

> In addition to her good work, Miss Snively was keenly interested in affairs of the world, in certain aspects of literature, and was particularly devoted to church and missionary work, so that the nurses trained by her were transformed from girls who were more or less crude to women with poise, thoroughness, independence and enterprise.[61]

Furthermore, this ideal nurse performed a humanitarian public service that was based on the service idea rather than on money. It is clear that most Canadian physicians preferred that nursing remain a spiritual vocation and not develop into a secular profession.

Graduate nurses did not participate in this ideological debate but rather focused their attention on practical matters. Issues relating to unemployment, working conditions for nurses, and the ideals of professionalism were discussed but the reality of the changing economic conditions demanded their attention. These rank-and-file nurses developed new initiatives to deal with the economic situation and supported each other in order to sustain their mutual survival. They also ensured that Canadians received quality nursing service and in so doing, secured a place for nursing service that would clearly enhance its role in society.

The Great Depression also had implications for public health nurses. The changing intellectual climate of the day produced a transformation in theories of public health. The <u>Canadian Public Health Journal</u> described this evolving concept as follows:

> Society has a basic responsibility for assuring, to all of its members, healthful conditions of housing and living, a reasonable degree of economic security, proper facilities for

curative and preventive medicine and adequate medical care – in fact the control, so far as means are known to science, of all environmental factors that affect physical and mental well-being.[62]

In order to fulfill this responsibility, society looked to public health nurses for assistance. This in turn lent further credence to the professional goals of nursing. Public health nurses received further encouragement and public support for their expanding role because their services could be provided more economically than those of a physician. The growing need resulted in a shortage of skilled public health nurses resulting in recruitment programs that emphasized their advanced education and increasing value to the community they served. These developments in public health nursing contributed to the creation of a permanent niche for nursing in Canadian society that would also support professionalism for nursing. The continued objections raised by members of the medical profession were met with strategies that alternated between cooperation and assertiveness. But the close relationship public health nurses had with their community mirrored that of the private duty nurses and garnered them the support they needed to survive opposition and the trials of the 1930s. Therefore, in many ways, the public health nurse exemplified the success of nursing's tenacity, determination, and commitment to the concept of professionalism during this difficult decade.

Given the depressed economic climate of the 1930s, it is not surprising that the health of the community was an important topic. Canadians agreed that during a time of financial stress, public health work was urgently needed and should be offered as a public service. Indeed, public health officials suggested that agencies, whether constituted on a statutory or a voluntary basis, should make every effort to meet the greater need experienced during a period of depression.[63] In all cases, the onus fell on the public health nurse. In the outpost, the public health nurse represented a hospital, a visiting nurse, and a public health nurse, all rolled into one practitioner. In the school, the public health nurse examined and taught the children prevention of disease.[64] In some provinces, public health nursing involved pre-natal work, infant welfare work, pre-school examination of children, health inspection of schools, education regarding Tuberculosis and Trachoma, home-nursing instruction, and communicable disease prevention. Little wonder that Ruby Simpson, a public health nurse in Saskatchewan, described the public health nurse as being:

> well-trained, experienced, adaptable, tactful and diplomatic, patient and persevering. She needs a keen sense of humour to carry her over many difficult places and a strong physique for the rigours of rural travel. A strong sense of the importance of her work and of the satisfaction in a difficult task well attempted, and at least a step made, toward the goal of all public health effort.[65]

As a result of this somewhat complex and expanding role of the public health nurse, she was accepted as an *essential* member of the public health forces of any community. In order to assist the modern public health nurse to adapt to this changing social order, the education of the public health nurses had to prepare them for what was becoming an expanding professional service.[66]

Despite such a demand, the number of nurses willing to work in public health did not expand with the role. Weir had recommended in the Survey that "the number of public health nurses in Canada should be doubled within the next five or ten years."[67] Elizabeth Smellie once again urged more cooperation between the schools of nursing and the public health agencies in order to expose student nurses to the advantages of working in public health. Public health nursing was presented in a positive and happy light, full of variety and always challenging. The Metropolitan Life Insurance Company advertisements painted the visiting nurse as the sole reason for the declining death rates from Tuberculosis, Influenza, Measles, Pneumonia, Whooping

Cough, Diphtheria, and Scarlet Fever.[68] Public health nurses, particularly those who worked in the isolated areas of northern and rural Canada, received international recognition.[69] In these isolated parts of Canada, nurses worked independently and since physicians tended to be few and far between, there was little rivalry or fear of competition.

This was not the case in the southern and urban parts of Canada. Here they encountered hostility from their colleagues. Ethel Cryderman, Central Supervisor of the Victorian Order of Nurses for Canada, advised them in the pages of The Canadian Nurse, to employ professional etiquette in order to maintain a cooperative relationship with the physicians. This professional etiquette was based on acknowledgment of the leadership of the medical profession. One strategy recommended was to encourage every pregnant woman to place herself under the care and supervision of a physician.[70] The public health nurse was also advised to cooperate with all community workers because:

> "good" public health nurses are those who do not annoy their co-workers but who, in spite of this, let me add, manage to make the fullest use of all community workers and their resources for the benefit of the families under their care.[71]

Although these relationships were always described as partnerships, giving them an egalitarian flavour, the ultimate goal of the partnership with the physician was "to give them the best service we can in each individual case and to report back to them continuously."[72] Indeed, the teaching that was accomplished in public health was not only directed toward sending patients to physicians but also to ensure that these patients were prepared to be "good patients."[73] Unfortunately this cooperative partnership always seemed to carry patronizing elements. For example, an American physician, R. Atwater, who was also the Executive secretary for the American Public Health Association, discussed "The Place of the Public Health Nurse in a Community Program" at the twenty-eighth annual meeting of the Canadian Public Health Association, in 1939. Atwater began by commenting on the fact that his topic was safe because most speakers would not "be expected to say anything revolutionary" about nursing service in the community. He viewed the public health nurse to be most important in the community but advised that his:

> counsel to all public health nurses was that they be very patient with the medical officers of health so that the physicians might understand the purposes of the other and mutually co-operate for the good of the service as well as for the good of the community.[74]

He delivered his address to the Public Health Nursing Section and the Section of Vital Statistics and Epidemiology that would influence his position. He concluded his remarks by encouraging "a cooperative understanding between nursing and other parts of the health enterprise" in order to "look forward with confidence to that which the future holds."

The close relationship public health nurses enjoyed with the community around them necessarily involved them in societal issues. Immigrants continued to be an issue for Canadians and public health nurses cooperated with physicians in debating the issue of the preservation of the race. Their participation, however, did not only occur at the level of discussion. Public health nurses continued to support ideas about eugenics that were also promoted by the physicians during this decade. The Canadian Nurse noted that a female physician attending a National Council of Women meeting "condemned the general sterilization of the mentally defective" but that the Council dropped the topic for the next few years, postponing any decision on the matter.[75] This cautious approach was common to most professions but the tacit agreement and proactive behaviour of nurses increased their interaction with the society around them. One fascinating example of this participation occurred on the prairies.

There was overwhelming support for the sexual sterilization activities that were approved by the Alberta Eugenics Board.[76] These sentiments received further support in the activities of the birth control movement established by a Kitchener businessman, A.R. Kaufman, in 1933. He hired women from across Canada to promote the use of birth control packages that he distributed through the philanthropy of his Parent's Information Bureau. Kaufman, a self-proclaimed eugenicist, successfully defended his activities in an Ontario court in 1936 and 1937, thus giving him the freedom to continue his fight for the betterment of the race.[77]

When the Wesley United Church in Calgary decided to establish the Family Planning Association in 1937, they hired a Kaufman nurse, Ann Hammill, as a consultant to assist in the promotion of birth control material. Hammill was paid $19.95 per month plus an additional $1.00 for every application for birth control that she sent to the Parent's Information Bureau in Kingston. The application incorporated a brief medical history of the client, home conditions and information relevant to birth control devices. Further information was available in English, Polish, Ukrainian, or French and all supplies were free of charge. She worked cooperatively with the Eugenics Board of Alberta and described them as "very helpful." In fact all of the "abnormal" cases were referred to the Board and for Hammill, abnormal meant families in which one or two children out of five or six had a physical deformity. This nurse was committed to her work. Indeed, for her, given the economic climate of the thirties, the government could not bear the cost of the many children who eventually became wards of the State.[78]

Sterilization was viewed as a path to racial improvement.[79] To avoid the risk of transmission of any negative racial characteristics to Canadian society, a medical examination of all immigrants was conducted prior to their departure for Canada. This was done to protect Canadians from the many communicable diseases identified with nationalities other than

British.[80] Success in this regard was reported by Dr. C.P. Brown to the Sixth Pacific Science Congress in 1939. He reported:

> During the past four years a total of 1,036 prospective immigrants were refused admission because of mental and physical defects brought to light by these examinations. This was at the rate of 18 per 1000 actual admissions. The efficiency of this service is evidenced by the fact that in the last four years only 31 individuals have been deported by virtue of conditions that pre-existed their arrival, this out of the many thousands who have made their homes in Canada over the past years.[81]

The support and cooperation public health nurses gave the philosophy of eugenics reflects the fundamentally important role they played within their communities. This also reveals their biases and the kind of attitudes they would have had to the very people they were trying to help.

This cooperation on the part of the public health nurses did not appear to be enough because they continued to encounter opposition from their medical colleagues in public health as well. For the physicians, the ideal nurse was difficult to find among those nurses involved in public health work. The medical profession expected the public health nurse to be the epitome of diplomacy and closely allied with the family physician. This was not always the case. One psychiatrist described the public health nurse as a negative, or harmful influence in the field of mental health.[82] Territorial fears in the area of public health are reflected in the following excerpt:

> It would be hardly the truth to say that all is well between the public health nursing service and the practising physician. There is an underlying resentment on the part of the doctor for what he believes to be an unwise encroachment on his individual relation with the family ... For he feels that in so much teaching the nurse is invading

his domain and that, comparatively, she is less well equiped[sic] for this work than he.[83]

In many instances, physicians viewed the public health nurse as inadequately prepared. Yet surprisingly, the same physicians fought against any improvements in the educational preparation of nurses during this period.

During the thirties, public health nurses carved out for themselves a secure place within Canadian society and in so doing, furthered professionalism for nursing. While efficiently fulfilling their role in the community, they encountered considerable opposition from the medical profession and employed collaboration and cooperation to appease the physicians. This position dictated the way in which all other issues were addressed as is evidenced in their support for eugenics and concerns about immigrants. They joined the medical profession and much of Canadian society in their concerns about eliminating the defective from Canadian stock. This intimate link to the medical profession also influenced how the public health nurses viewed the role they played in the delivery of health services in the community. Emphasis was always placed on the physician as the supervisor of all cases and one who must be kept informed at all times. The public health nurses would have followed through on this as much as possible but the more isolated their place of work was, the less likely it would be that this would occur. In spite of the apparent subservience of these public health nurses to the medical profession, the nurses did improve their educational preparation and this further enhanced their value to the community. Furthermore, the subservient role was transitory and appeared to be simply a strategy to pacify any opposition that emerged.

The tensions that existed between nursing and medicine resulted in some considerable confusion for the Canadian public. The shortage of financial resources generated criticism of the nurses' salary requirements. Weir commented early in 1932, that a considerable number of people believed that the nursing profession was becoming commercialized and that it was losing the personal touch and the so-called Florence Nightingale spirit.[84] The public wanted a nurse to be self-sacrificing and public-spirited and expressed a growing concern regarding the high cost of medical care. Indeed, many Canadians believed that people of moderate means could not afford to be sick.[85] A minority supported the nurse's right to an adequate salary and benefits but this support was weak.[86] The public did value nursing service and admitted to making use of it when necessary but appeared to be confused when it was necessary to place any monetary value on that service.

In many respects nurses had gained in the eyes of the public but the occasional bout of confusion generated negativity as well. The professional hygienic expert of the twenties was now criticized for that role. One literary figure, E.J. Pratt, noted that "nursing falls into three classifications: the good, the bad and the indifferent." His far from indifferent opinion of a nurse emphasized the nurse's need to examine, polish, and clean up her patients both internally and externally.[87] The picture that accompanied this poem depicted a dark, stern, and angry woman. The dark image of the nurse connected her to the gloominess of the period.

Romantic depictions of nurses were present in numerous novels, plays, and movies. Many novels, published in serial form in magazines, involved romance with a physician and self-denial on the part of the nurse and always ended happily. The plays contributed to this image in their portrayal of the nurse as "gay, humorous, lovely and brave all at once."[88] The same was true in movies. One nurse pointed out the morals of a recent popular movie involving a nurse:

> The story is about a nurse who is first shown getting her training at a hospital, fighting with internes[sic] and assisting at important operations ... It is through her struggle

with the villains – aided, of course, by a young bootlegger, who is fond of her – that everything turns out happily at the end. And if any readers find the union of a nurse and a bootlegger distasteful, they must remember that the nurse reformed the bootlegger, thereby holding up the standards of the profession![89]

Confusion dominated nursing developments during the thirties. The energetic intellectual climate and the publication of the "Weir Report" provided nursing with an opportunity to pursue its professional goals in spite of the stormy economic situation. The Depression clearly created problems for nursing, but nurses employed skilful tactics to enable the profession to "weather the storm." Nursing leaders worked towards advancing and standardizing nursing education. Although graduate nurses and public health nurses spent some of their time simply reacting to the difficulties they encountered, the nursing skill they provided ensured that nursing service became a valued commodity in both the hospital and the community. The close interaction that nurses experienced with the society around them gave them the self-confidence to withstand the opposition dispensed by the medical profession while also involving them more closely with societal issues of the day. This interassociation undoubtedly exposed nursing to criticism from some segments of society, especially physicians. Statements by the medical profession only added to the unsettling situation. Still, taken altogether, nurses demonstrated not only their ability to "weather the storm" but even to have taken a few more important steps towards their goal of professional status.

By the close of the thirties, Canadian nursing had achieved some considerable success in terms of the first three criteria of professionalism: post-secondary education, a certification test, and a degree of self-regulation. Their success was evident on the eve of this decade when nurses were invited to participate in a meeting of the International Hospital Association in Toronto, in 1939. Unfortunately, Germany invaded Poland and war was declared thus diminishing the size and impact of the meeting. Wartime service once again would present opportunities for nurses to prove their professional worth.

CHAPTER FOUR NOTES

[1] "Hundreds in Throng to Honor Miss Dyke," The Toronto Daily Star, May 6, 1933.

[2] David Naylor, Private Practice, Public Payment: Canadian Medicine and the Politics of Health Insurance, 191101966, (Kingston: McGill-Queen's University Press, 1986), pp. 67, 112, 113. The health insurance fund was not yet in existence but was proposed as a modest form of insurance.

[3] For a fuller discussion see John Herd Thompson and Allen Seager, Canada 1922-1939.

[4] H.Blair Neatby, The Politics of Chaos: Canada in the Thirties, (Toronto: Macmillan of Canada, 1972), pp. 19-187.

[5] Doug Owram, The Government Generation, p. 190.

[6] Paul Axelrod, Making a Middle Class: Student Life in English Canada During the Thirties, (Montreal: McGill-Queen's UP, 1990), p. 91.

[7] Mary Kinnear, Margaret McWilliams: An Interwar Feminist, (Montreal: McGill-Queens' University Press, 1991), p. 160.

[8] G.M.Weir, Survey of Nursing Education in Canada, (Toronto: University of Toronto Press, 1932), p. 5, 65.

[9] Ibid, p. 86..

[10] Browne, Jean E., "The Forgotten Nurse," CN, Vol. XXVII, No.12, December 1931, pp. 621,622.

[11] "The Survey East and West," CN, Vol. XXIX, No. 6, June 1933, p. 295, 296.

[12] The Hon. Vincent Massey, "The Public and the Survey," Canadian Nurses' Association Biennial Meeting, Saint John, N.B., June 21, 1932, OCHA and Reba Riddell, "Nurses and Nursing," The Canadian Forum, Vol. 13, 1933/34, pp. 9,10.

[13] George Weir, Survey, pp. 392,393.

[14] Russell, E. Kathleen, "A Recent Gift for a Nursing School," Canadian Public Health Journal (CPHJ), Vol. 24, No.1, January 1933, p.43. Also noted in "A Backward Glance at the Toronto Hospital Meetings," TNHR, November, 1939, p.436.

[15] Carpenter, Helen, A Divine Discontent: Edith Kathleen Russell: Reforming Educator, (Toronto: University of Toronto Press, 1982), pp.19,20. For further information regarding university education for

nurses see Rondalyn Kirkwood's unpublished Ph.D. Dissertation, "The Development of University Education in Canada, 1920-1975: Two Case Studies," 1988.

[16] George Weir, Survey, p. 393.

[17] "Ryerson to Falconer," November 12, 1930, A67-0007/127B, UTA.

[18] "Reports of the Committee," 1934-1939, A73-0053/06/02, UTA.

[19] Lindeburgh Marion, "The McGill School for Graduate Nurses," CN, Vol. XXXIV, No.6, June 1938, p. 302.

[20] Lindeburgh, "McGill School," CN, Vol. XXXIV, no.6, June 1938, p. 302.

[21] Canadian Nurses Association, Proposed Curriculum for Schools of Nursing in Canada, (Montreal: Canadian Nurses Association, 1936), p. 9.

[22] Jean S. Wilson, "Report of Executive Secretary June 1934," p.2, CNAA.

[23] Ruby Simpson, "Thirty Years of Growth," CN, Vol. XXXIV, No. 8, August 1938, p. 416.

[24] Ethel Johns, "The Editor's Desk," CN, Vol. XXXII, No.12, December 1936, p. 551.

[25] Mary M. Roberts, "Current Events and Trends in Nursing," CN, Vol. XXV, No.1, January 1939, p. 13.

[26] Doug Owram, The Government Generation, p. 240, 242, 252.

[27] Ruby Simpson et al., "A Submission to the Royal Commission on Dominion-Provincial Relations," CN, Vol. XXXIV, No.7, July 1938, p. 371, 373, 374.

[28] J.H. Elliot, "Nursing Service in the Community - The Point of View of the Physician," CLP, October, 1933, p. 111.

[29] Basil C. MacLean, "Nurses - What Next?," CN, Vol. XXXII, No.11, November 1936, pp. 497-506.

[30] Madge Thurlow Macklin, "Five o'clock in the Morning," CN, Vol. XXXIII, No.7, July 1937, pp. 319-322.

[31] Edith Henry audiotaped interview. According to Henry, graduate nurses were labelled as "Private Duty" nurses, they were often employed within the hospital setting. Henry was a graduate of the Calgary General Hospital and later Director of Nursing in that facility.

[32] See David H. Gibson, "The Nursing Depression: A Doctor Speaks Out," TNHR, Vol. 88, No.2, pp. 179-181 and Agnes Ruth Riddles, "A Nurse Speaks," TNHR, Vol. 88, No.2, p. 185 and Grace Rowan, "The Crisis in Private Nursing," CN, Vol. XXIX, no.12, December 1933, p. 645.

[33] Rowan, pp. 646-647.

[34] Jean E. Browne, "Correspondence," CN, Vol. XXXII, No.12, December 1936, p. 552.

[35] Janet M. Geister, "We Say It Again," TNHR, February, 1939, pp. 119-122.

[36] "Inquiring Reporter," TNHR, February, 1939, p. 123.

[37] "From a Private Duty Nurses' Diary," CN, Vol. XXVII, No.2, February 1931, p. 86.

[38] "Private Duty Nurses Forum," CN, Vol. XXX, No.7, July 1934, p. 322.

[39] "Nursing in Canada," (CLP), Vol. 83, No.6, December 1934, p. 164.

[40] "Department of Private Duty Nursing: What Do You Think About It?," CN, Vol. XXXI, No.10, October 1935, p. 450.

[41] Florence Dewey, "Department of Private Duty Nursing: The Eight Hour day," CN, Vol. XXXI, No.5, May 1935, pp. 216-218.

[42] "Department of Private Duty Nursing: What Do You Think About It?," CN, Vol. XXXI, No.6, June 1935, p. 267 and "Department of Private Duty Nursing: What Do You Think About It?," CN, Vol. XXXI, No.7, July 1935, p. 311.

[43] M.J. Leslie, "How We Got the Eight-Hour Day," CN, Vol. XXXIII, No.1, January 1937, pp. 28-29. See also "Department of Private Duty Nursing: Where Do We Stand," CN, Vol. XXXI, No.9, September 1935, pp. 409-413, and "Department of Private Duty Nursing: It Can Be Done!," CN, Vol. XXXII, No.6, June 1936, pp. 258-260.

[44] "The Right to Live," CN, Vol. XXXII, No.2, February 1936, p. 65.

[45] Jo Ann Whittaker, "The Comox Nurses Strike of 1939," B.C. Historical News, 22/4, 1989, p. 20.

[46] "The Calgary Experiment," CN, Vol. XXX, No.11, November 1934, p. 516.

[47] "Annual General Meeting of the AARN," 1938, AARN Official Minutes - Council, Vol. 4, p. 451, AARNA.

[48] AARN Annual Reports of the Secretary, 1927-1943, p. 15. AARNA.

[49] "Report of Unemployment Among Nurses in Alberta," CN, Vol. XXVIII, No.6, June 1932, p. 305.

[50] "An Improvised Incubator," CN, Vol. XXXI, No.1, January 1935, p. 17.

[51] Isabel Irvine, "Nursing on the Prairies," p. 6, OCHA.

[52] Edith Young, "Highlights of," p. 4.

[53] Isabel MacIntosh, "Nursing Service from the Standpoint of the Nurse," CN, Vol. XXVI, No.7, July 1930, p. 354, 356.

[54] "Techniques for the Selection of Students," TNHR, Vol. 88, No.3, March 1932, p. 321.

[55] Edith F. Naylor, "Life Offered Up," CN, Vol. XXXII, No.3, March 1936, p. 106. The debate continued in CN, Vol. XXXII, No.4, April 1936, pp. 160-161.

[56] "Are You a Good Nurse?," CN, Vol. XXXIV, No.1, January 1938, pp. 31-32.

[57] Catherine de Nully Fraser, "Where are We Drifting?," CN, Vol. XXVII, No.8, August 1931, p. 424.

[58] Phyllis Gilbert, "Why You Should Belong," CN, Vol. XXXII, No.4, April 1936, p. 157.

[59] Jean S. Wilson, "Military Service," CN, Vol. XXXV, No.9, September 1939, p. 562 and Ethel Johns, "Guarding the Flame," CN, Vol. XXXV, No.9, September 1939, p. 562.

[60] G. Stewart Cameron, "A Word of Counsel," CN, Vol. XXXII, No.3, March 1936, pp. 101-102.

[61] "The Canadian Nightingale," CLP, January, 1934, p. 4.

[62] "The Changing Concept of Public Health," CPHJ, Vol. 27, No.1, January 1936, p. 19.

[63] "Editorial," CPHJ, Vol. 23, No.3, March 1932, p. 140.

[64] Doris C. Jackson, "The Outpost and Health Teaching," CPHJ, Vol. 21, No.6, June 1930, pp. 296-299 and Mary Millman, "Special Classes as a Factor in Health," CPHJ, Vol. 21, No.7, July 1930, pp. 355-357.

[65] Ruby M. Simpson, "Public Health Nursing in Saskatchewan," CPHJ, Vol. 22, No.3, March 1931, pp. 130-134.

[66] Marion Lindeburgh, "The Educational Objective of Public Health Nursing," CPHJ, Vol. 25, No.9, September 1934, pp. 443-447.

[67] George Weir, Survey, p. 143.

[68] "Why Canada is Healthier...," CPHJ, Vol. 30, No.11, November 1939.

[69] Leslie Bell, "Pioneer Health Work in Canada," TNHR, Vol. 89, No.6, pp. 643-647.

[70] Ethel Cryderman, "The Relationship of the Visiting Nurse to the Medical Profession," CN, Vol. XXVI, No.6, June 1930, pp. 315-316 and M.S. Taylor, "The Public Health Nurse - Her Work in Relation to Maternal Mortality," CPHJ, Vol. 21, No.8, July 1930, pp. 349-351.

[71] Mary S. Mathewson, "Public Health Nursing," CPHJ, Vol. 26, No.1, January 1935, pp. 47-49.

[72] Alma C. Haupt, "Partnership in Public Health Nursing," CPHJ, Vol. 27, No.6, June 1936, p. 273.

[73] Floyd S. Winslow, "Partners in Public Health," CN, Vol. XXXIII, No.2, February 1937, p. 74.

[74] Reginald M. Atwater, "The Place of the Public Health Nurse in a Community Program," CPHJ. Vol. 30, No.5, June 1939, p. 279.

[75] Jennie M. Allen, "National Council of Women in Canada," CN, Vol. XXVI, No.11, November 1930, p. 588.

[76] For further discussion of this topic see Angus McLaren, Our Own Master Race: Eugenics in Canada, 1885-1945, (Toronto: McClelland & Stewart, 1990) and Ian H. Clarke, "Public Provisions for the Mentally Ill in Alberta, 1907-1936," Unpublished MA Thesis, University of Calgary, 1973 and R.R. MacLean & E.J. Kibblewhite, "Sexual Sterilization in Alberta," CPHJ, Vol. 28, No.12, December 1937.

[77] Angus McLaren, Master Race. p. 77.

[78] Audiotaped interview with Ann Hammill conducted by Patty White in Calgary, 1984.

[79] C.B. Farrar, "Editorial," CPHJ, vol. 32, no.1, January 1931, p. 93.

[80] F.W. Jackson, "Racial Origin in Relation to Public Health Activities," CPHJ, Vol. 22, No.6, June 1931, pp. 311-316.

[81] C.P. Brown, "The Present Status of Health in Canada," p. 9, Brown, C.P. Articles 1938-1939, RG29, Volume 2355, NAC. Also see Barbara Roberts, Whence They Came: Deportation from Canada 1900-1935, (Ottawa: Ottawa University Press, 1988).

[82] W.T.B. Mitchell, "The Psychiatrist Looks at Public Health Nursing," CPHJ, Vol. 23, No.10, October 1932, pp. 455-459.

[83] A.M. Jeffrey, "The Private Physician Looks at Public Health Nursing," CPHJ, Vol. 23, No.10, October 1932, pp. 462-463.

[84] George Weir, "The Public and the Nurse," CN, Vol. XXVI, No.9, September 1930, p. 494.

[85] Frederick L. Collins, "The High Cost of Being Sick," LHJ, October 1930, pp. 16,17,82.

[86] Reba Riddell, "Nurses and Nursing," CF, Vol. 13, 1933/34, pp. 9-10.

[87] E.J. Pratt, "To Angelina, An Old Nurse," CF, Vol. 11, 1931/32, p. 141.

[88] "Private Duty: A Novel of Love and Conflict with a Life Devoted to Service," LHJ, Vol. 52:1935 to Vol. 53:1936.

[89] Lillian Sabine, "The Nurse in Current Drama," TNHR, Vol. 87, No.6, December 1931, p. 758.

Chapter Five

SUPPLY, DEMAND, ECONOMICS AND PROFESSIONALISM: WORLD WAR II

Canadian nurses survived the hardships of the Depression and became of greater value to Canada in the war years. In the process, nursing continued to distance itself from the concept of vocation and moved towards the goal of secular profession. This course of events was maintained by virtue of the fact that nursing mirrored what was happening in society at large. Both groups had common goals, the most important being to support Canada's war effort. This, in turn, meant a shortage of nurses and a demand for their essential services, resulting in an advance of nursing's professional cause. But at the same time, the growing involvement of the public-at-large, most often politicians, with nursing during the war years meant that these outsiders dictated developments in nursing, often undermining the professional vision of the nursing leaders. On the other hand, nursing gained from this interference as well, in that government grants in support of nursing education materialized. Nursing, therefore, would meet the service criteria of professionalism and their service received further acknowledgement through these government funds.

The path to professionalism, however, was not entirely smooth during this period. The growing unrest that percolated among nurses themselves was in sharp contrast to the collegial encounter nurses had with their medical associates. Similarly, the old image of the nurse as a moral guardian resurfaced by the close of the war. Overall, nurses emerged from the Second World War as a group of respected professionals who had successfully met society's expectations. The willingness of Canadian nurses to join all Canadians in the war effort was a fundamental component in the success they attained.

The outbreak of World War Two united most Canadians in support of Britain and the war effort. Indeed, the Canadian military effort in the Second World War was the largest of any secondary power. Canadians not only participated overseas but gave their unconditional support at home as well. They accepted the far-reaching and severe constraints placed upon them and met all the demands of the government. All levels of Canadian society supported and financed the war through the Victory Bond campaigns. Hardships aside, historian Kenneth McNaught concludes that "the accumulation of wealth in many forms outstripped by far what was spent on the war effort" indeed, "the impulse given by the war to Canadian economic growth carried the country into the ranks of the industrialized states."[1] Furthermore, most Canadians adapted to these wartime conditions enthusiastically and willingly.

Although the participation of women in Canada's war effort did nothing to change the traditional roles or stereotypes associated with "women's work," to some extent the war redistributed them from low-paying work in trade and domestic service into better-paying factory work. But, as historian Ruth Roach Pierson points out, their most outstanding contribution was in terms of their unpaid work in the home and in their communities.[2]

One result of the war effort was the centralization of power. The hardships of the Depression had led many Canadians to believe that mass unemployment was avoidable if the central government controlled the fiscal and monetary policy. This centralist position was enhanced when the demands of war gave Ottawa direct responsibility for the nation's labour force. Opinion polls revealed that the majority of Canadians agreed with this move. This was probably due to the fact that most Canadians looked to Ottawa for material security during the war, fearing otherwise a return to the depressed economic times of the thirties. Ottawa responded by imposing regulations – regulations that affected all goods and services. Federal intervention achieved the desired goal that meant even greater intrusion from the central government. Thanks to the war effort and the increased demand of government, the nation moved from underemployment to full employment; the workforce was mobilized; serious inflation avoided; living standards improved; and a more equitable distribution of burdens and benefits achieved.[3]

Within Canada, the unity that resulted from the war effort contributed to a shift in the balance of power from the provinces to the federal government. The result was a wartime government that was interventionist, centralist, and in a position to take authoritative social measures.[4] This move was reinforced by the recommendations of the Report on Dominion-Provincial Relations, usually known as the Rowell-Sirois Report, issued in 1940. The acceptance of the Rowell-Sirois Commission's recommendations ensured that the state would become more involved in the lives of the public. Indeed, historian Doug Owram has concluded that "the majority of the intellectual community, the needs of modern society, and the public mood dictated that the state continue to expand its role."[5] The war offered the federal government many opportunities to fulfill this expectation. In doing so, the interventionist role snowballed on many levels. This expanded role encompassed investigations into nursing as well. Consequently, a total of four surveys of nursing were done between 1941 and 1946 by either provincial or federal governments.

What should be the role of nurses in the war effort? This was the overarching question of the Canadian Nurses Association's Biennial Meeting held in Calgary, in 1940. Six months earlier the Canadian Nurses Association had held an Executive Meeting and agreed to write Prime Minister Mackenzie King to convey to him their assurance that the Canadian Nurses Association, and all nine provincial associations, loyally supported the federal government.[6] They had also promised The Canadian Red Cross Society War Council that members of the nursing profession in Canada were ready and willing to render any national service requested of them.[7] Now they were meeting to discuss how best to fulfill this promise. Elizabeth Smellie, Matron-in-Chief, presided over one key session that addressed "nurses and nursing at home and abroad in time of war." The purpose of the panel and the ensuing debate was to plan for a new recruitment campaign. In one other closely related session, the speaker "shed light on many of our present difficulties."[8] Clearly, nurses considered themselves to be an integral part of Canadian society and were eager to fulfill demands made on them during this time of crisis.

To encourage military service, the Association published correspondence received from nurses who were already overseas. Most letters contained very little factual data but presented attractive narrative pictures to encourage enlistment. One nurse wrote:

> Will you please thank all those good friends of mine who combined to send me such a lovely and generous Christmas parcel. We have been constantly on the move – clearing up and making habitable one lot of billets after another – and learning the ways of one military hospital after another. I do not know where we are going, or where I shall be sleeping two nights from now! But wherever we go we shall try and do what is required of us with all our hearts and wills.[9]

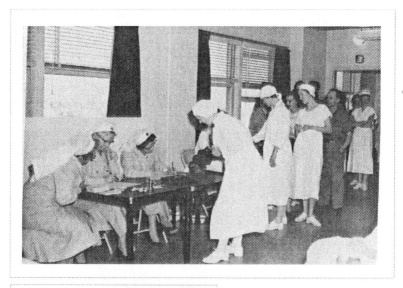

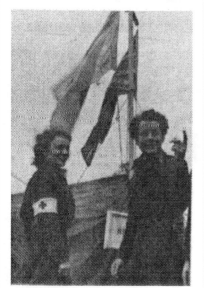

Canadian Nurses during WWII.

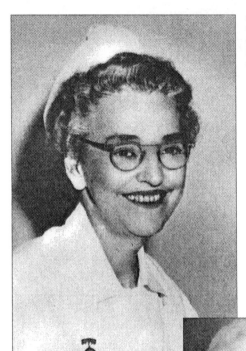

Gertrude Hall was asked by the Calgary General Hospital to resolve staffing difficulties faced by the hospital; all of the nurses had walked off the job.

Edith Kathleen Russell, Director of the School of Nursing at the University of Toronto, oversaw the implementation of the first independent baccalaureate degree program. (Both photos courtesy Helen K. Mussallem Library)

146

This nurse presented her experience as a much-anticipated adventure, but others were more subdued:

> Imagine my surprise (and almost disgust) to receive a phone call on Thursday, August 31, asking me to report for duty at 2 a.m.! I couldn't get over it, and felt very much the martyr I am afraid, staying up all night in a first aid post ... There were half-a-dozen of us there, to lay casualties out on the floor if they came to us.[10]

In spite of the fact that both of these letters imparted a certain routinization of the impact of the war on nurses, they did attract nurses by the prospect of adventure.

Military nursing was presented as more than just adventure. The Canadian Nurse presented such nursing as exciting in terms of the opportunity it offered to be a part of scientific advances. Nurses were told that only those nurses who were highly skilled and knowledgeable should serve overseas because the injuries and conditions being treated were becoming increasingly complex. Surgeries were increasing and becoming very specialized therefore, any assistance would require advanced nursing skill to deal with the dressings. Furthermore, "up-to-date" knowledge had become indispensable to nurse in this field. As Fanny C. Munroe, Superintendent of Nurses at the Royal Victoria Hospital in Montreal, noted:

> Preparation should ... be professional, moral, [and] mental. A greater physical courage is needed, as no one will be safe, and everyone must be willing and able to work, although afraid. Skill and speed, developed through an experience of hard work will be essential – a preparation almost all nurses have had, and ability to hold steady in a new and difficult situation, and judgment such that you see the important thing in each new problem.[11]

Popular magazines with photographs of nursing sisters performing a variety of functions both at home and abroad also publicized the importance of nursing overseas.[12]

The publicity paid off. Canadian nurses flocked to join. In fact, the numbers were so great that Elizabeth Smellie, Matron-in-Chief of the World War II Army Medical Corps, visited a number of Canadian hospitals to discourage enlistment and to remind nurses that services were needed at home as well. Elizabeth Laurie Smellie was on leave from her job as Chief Superintendent of the VON and became the first Canadian woman to achieve the rank of Colonel. She also organized the Canadian Women's Army Corps. Retired public health nurses easily recall their meetings with Smellie during which she refused to accept their applications to join the medical corps.[13]

The war effort strained nursing resources at home to the limit. In 1941, there were a total of 26,473 graduate nurses in Canada, 8,000 of whom were associated with the Medical Corps. Approximately 4,000 nurses were required for 34 overseas military hospitals, 60 domestic military hospitals and 2 hospital ships. The remaining 22,000 nurses were expected to deliver nursing service to the civilian population spread across the country. Nursing, therefore, became an indispensable service to a nation at war – a situation that would prove to be of immeasurable advantage to nursing's quest for professionalism.

Maintaining a healthy population became a high priority of the government during the war effort. The government developed programs to build a positive, virile, healthy Canadian population that would be able to support the Canadian war effort. This notion represented a change in the goal of health care services. As one physician observed:

> In the past, we were inclined to think of the international health front in terms of repressive measures – quarantines and restrictions to keep disease from entering our respective national boundaries. Today we collaborate for international

health through pooling the health, medical and research brains of each nation to win war.[14]

The health of the family was a fundamentally important component, if the war was to be won. To this end, all nurses, particularly public health nurses, assisted the family to achieve maximum health and independence through counselling and health teaching. The accepted theory was that solidarity of the family was essential to maintain the morale of the father who had enlisted to defend his country.[15]

The important role given the nurse at home was equalled overseas where the nurse often worked in isolated situations. One narrative in the publication <u>Canada At War</u> noted:

> In the case of a crash or accident, the Air Force Nurse must be self-sufficient in a fashion rarely encountered in the other services. The Medical Officer will be at the scene of the crash, and the nurse must direct all activity in the hospital and be certain that everything is in readiness when he arrives with the patients. She has no matron or supervisor to whom she can appeal, and she must keep her assistants from becoming alarmed and excited.[16]

Clearly, for nursing to fulfill these roles both at home and overseas would place pressure on existing nursing resources.

Nursing developments, therefore, emerged out of recruitment initiatives taken to fulfill the growing demand for nursing services. Nursing leaders directed publicity campaigns that presented nursing as an attractive alternative to competing career opportunities. Increasing career choices for women in conjunction with the ongoing debate regarding women working at all, presented obstacles to recruitment, particularly for those women who were married with children.[17] Advances in nursing were rooted in the realization that their services had become a much-needed commodity, which in turn, underlined their importance to the community.

General duty nurses, both married and retired, were invited to return to active service. In Alberta, for example, Summer School Courses were offered to "all nurses registered in their respective provinces for 1943 who have practised their profession at some-time during the past ten years." Alberta also granted Wartime, or Temporary permits following the completion of a refresher course, to married and inactive nurses to help with the shortage of trained staff in civilian hospitals.[18] Indeed, the president of the Alberta Association of Registered Nurses told nurses residing in that province:

> You must decide where your work lies, and where your responsibility rests as a nurse and a patriotic citizen in a country suffering the duress of war. May you consider it carefully! May I remind you, too, that you are in the world, not in the profession of nursing only. You have a grave responsibility to the State, not only to give your professional service, but your will to keep informed and to be intelligently critical, so that you may add your voice to the plans for a better Canada.[19]

Nurses responded to calls such as this. Some of those whose children were grown returned to nursing, took the refresher course, and remained in the profession until retirement forced them to leave.

Provincial associations established publicity committees across Canada "to stimulate and encourage the attention of high school students to the opportunities of nursing."[20] Nursing leaders believed that to mobilize nursing at this point was to take advantage of the great opportunity the war afforded nursing to increase its usefulness. More importantly, the educational preparation that applicants would receive was described as scientific in such a way that it would equip the student with expert knowledge that would prepare her for work in a multitude of areas. The unity between the national and the provincial organizations that was apparent in these promotional efforts reinforced the public's positive perception of nursing and highlighted the fact that professional nursing was indispensable to the health and welfare of the community. The public became more informed about nurses, nursing, and nursing concerns.[21]

The national association decided to make more effective use of publicity in the recruitment campaigns because it had become apparent that many women were more attracted to industrial work than to nursing. In 1942, the Canadian Nurses Association investigated the entire area of publicity and concluded "successful distributors of publicity must be well versed in the subject to be publicized, in the tactics of camouflage, and other publicity techniques, and must be enthusiastic and consistently persistent."[22] This advertising material was sent to all Canadian newspapers. Free publicity was obtained from the <u>Canadian Press</u>, the <u>Canadian Home Journal</u>, <u>Chatelaine</u>, and the Canadian Broadcasting Corporation. All available popular communication techniques were utilized in that brochures, booklets, pamphlets and film promoted the indispensability of the nursing profession.

The Canadian Nurses Association admitted that this was a departure from their usual behaviour. Indeed, Kathleen W. Ellis, Emergency Nursing Advisor, made the following observation in <u>The Canadian Nurse</u>:

> Have not most nurses been prone to hide their lights under bushels and to shun newspaper reporters as potential sources of danger better avoided than explored? Now the Canadian Nurses Association has gone to seek publicity through the press, radio, and even the movies. Could some of our more discreet predecessors have believed it - and yet so it is.[23]

Much of the promotional material presented nurses as playing a fundamental role in the three key areas: curative, preventive, and health promotion. As one publication noted, the nurse had "gradually grown into a position of great responsibility in the community as a teacher of good health practices as well as the long-established Angel of Mercy in remedial nursing." The advertisements publicized the Victorian Order of Nurses in articles such as "Call the V.O.N...." Each area of nursing was presented as having a "glorious past and a rewarding future" and "a career for a girl with a courageous and sympathetic heart."[24]

Unfortunately, the shortage continued. The publicity campaign met with limited success in terms of recruitment, but great success in terms of informing the Canadian public of the importance of nursing. This increased awareness in turn advanced nursing as a profession.

Indeed, in the war years, nurses reported that they were treated with more respect.[25] The respectability of nursing was publicized in order to make the profession more attractive. This was reflected in the lengthy coverage given nursing in the important publication, <u>The Modern Hospital</u>. <u>The Canadian Nurse</u> reported that twenty-six pages were devoted to nursing service and nursing education in that journal. Although the article identified problems, it also gave proof positive that hospital administrators in high places were no longer taking nursing service for granted but were beginning to understand the importance of fostering and conserving it.[26] Married nurses who had returned to the profession wrote testimonials. One of them noted that:

> I feel that it is bracing to escape from the housekeeping and homemaking grooves into which I had settled and while there are two definite adjustments to be made each day – that of becoming professionally-minded, and then, domestically-minded – yet these are made more or less unconsciously.[27]

The life of a private duty nurse, previously described as least-desirable, was now reported to be most rewarding because it offered the best opportunities for the nurse to make use of all of her ability in the delivery of nursing care.[28]

Similar developments faced those nurses involved in public health. The outbreak of the war exacerbated the pre-war shortage and challenged the ingenuity of these nurses to deliver their service with fewer resources. The primary concern for public health nurses was not to lose people and services to the war effort. They feared that this could lead to an overtaxing of resources that would in turn, result in the increasing occurrence of sickness and death among infants and children.

The Canadian Nurses Association decided to cooperate in a survey of nursing resources. In 1942, the association appointed K.W. Ellis to the position of Emergency Nursing Advisor to investigate the entire nursing situation. She worked in conjunction with the Canadian Medical Procurement and Assignment Board, which included representatives from all groups involved in the delivery of health services in Canada. At the same time, the National Selective Service considered the advisability of conducting a registration of all graduate nurses.[29] One year later:

> Under a compulsory registration procedure conducted by the National Selective Service, all graduate nurses, active or inactive, married or single, were required to register with the Selective Service. The only exceptions were those graduate nurses serving in the armed forces.[30]

Out of this registration procedure came the decision that no nurse would be accepted for permanent or temporary national service unless she was registered in the province from which she applied.[31] Such government support would appear to confer legitimacy to nursing in Canada and would validate the efforts of the national organization. The results of the Survey, however, identified an acute shortage of general duty nurses. Indeed, this state of affairs persisted throughout the forties.

The ongoing shortage galvanized government intervention and the federal government allocated funds to support nursing education designed to assist and encourage young women to join the profession. The first annual grant to the Canadian Nurses Association in 1942 was $115,000.00, and this was increased to $250,000.00 in 1943 and in fact, continued for the duration of the war. The grants were to cover education, recruitment, and administration of the wartime program. The importance of the maintenance of the health of the public was reflected in the fact that public health nurses in Canada received twenty-five of the forty-five bursaries contained in one of these annual grants. These grants not only brought outside intervention through the accountability associated with government funding, but this funding support brought further recognition by the state too.[32] It is true that the grants were simply to alleviate the current nursing shortages, but many nurses viewed them as monetary rewards for the patriotic zeal with which nurses responded to the appeal for their services. In any event, the grants demonstrated an acknowledgment of the indispensability of nursing service.

The grants were in response to a Canadian Nurses Association appeal to the government for aid. The situation had become urgent if the provision of adequate national nursing service was to be met. Nursing leaders considered the grants to be recognition of nursing's contribution to national service. The funds were to be used for:

(a) Administration

(b) Direct assistance to schools of nursing to provide for increased registration

(c) Bursaries to enable graduate nurses to take post-graduate work

(d) Direct assistance to schools and departments of nursing in universities and public health organizations in order to extend their teaching facilities.[33]

The Canadian Nurses Association administered and accounted for all of the federal funds in a professional and reliable manner, thus adding to their professional image. As a result of these events, nurses interacted more with the government and with Canadians and became more self-confident.

The government grants not only assisted in the recruitment of nurses but also supported another ongoing concern for nursing leaders: nursing education. In the midst of a shortage of nurses, how could this problem be solved without compromising the standards already established for nursing education? Not surprisingly, given the sustained efforts of nursing educators over the years, they did not compromise their vision. Their endeavours continued to focus on the need for education as the ideal of nursing preparation, not apprenticeship-training. The task, however, was made more difficult in that it was attempted during a period in which the public demand for nurses escalated daily. Nonetheless, local initiatives did demonstrate progress in this regard, progress that advanced the cause of professionalism.

Kathleen Russell of the University of Toronto continued her crusade to further university education of nurses. In 1942, with the financial support of the Rockefeller Foundation and the University of Toronto, the university Senate approved her proposal for a degree program in nursing. As she noted in her Annual Report:

> The school is now in a position to turn to the claims of a degree course, which claims have become rather pressing because of the rapid developments in degree work both in our University and in many other Canadian institutions. This School now accepts the fact that the trend toward new degrees has been established beyond argument from any one single professional group; that, apparently, worthy standards can be set up and maintained; and most pertinent of all, that professional education in our own field of nursing

may be strengthened greatly by the proper use of this type of university work.[34]

Russell's goal was to provide professional preparation in nursing in combination with a broad liberal education that would serve the professional educational needs of nursing.

Russell wanted to prepare future leaders in nursing in teaching, hospital administration, nursing schools, and public health. In order to accomplish this goal, she added one year to the program to allow more time for professional and academic content.[35] As a result, the program changed in 1946 from a four to a five-year program and Russell discontinued the Basic, or Diploma Program that had been established in 1933. Russell identified a need for two levels of nursing expertise, one was leadership and the other was in clinical work. While the Canadian Nurses Association supported this completely, nurses across Canada required convincing.[36]

Canadians accepted progress in the education of public health nurses more readily. Society generally considered the role of the public health nurse to be essentially that of a teacher who was adequately prepared to translate the language of the scientific workers, or health care professionals, into the language of the ordinary citizen. In order to perform this function, the public health nurse required the special training contained in a recognized course in public health nursing.[37] In 1943, the minimum standard for employment in public health nursing was set as a nursing diploma plus at least one year of special preparation in public health nursing.[38] As early as 1941, the public health nurse was viewed as a "leader" in her community and the advanced educational and employment standards demanded of her only enhanced her professional status.[39]

Nonetheless, advances in general nursing education were inconsistent. Although some universities offered professional education, hospital schools continued to "train" nurses. The pressure of the war moved nursing leaders to investigate the feasibility of a shorter course of instruction as an emergency war measure. A "Canadian War Course" was considered in 1941 but not dealt with directly. Much debate regarding the need for a truly independent nursing school ensued. It was then determined that if the nursing school was totally independent of the hospital both financially and administratively, a professional nurse could be educated in two years.[40] Nursing had made significant strides but support for this innovative idea was not forthcoming until after the war.

In spite of the fact that the demand for nursing service had grown, working conditions had not improved. In 1943, therefore, the increasing popularity of trade unions moved the Canadian Nurses Association to form a Labour Relations Committee. It was formed "in response to the expressed need of some of the provincial associations, including British Columbia, for a national policy statement on nurse-trade union relationships."[41] The nursing profession had the support of most Canadians and could afford to be assertive. Prominent individuals such as Charlotte Whitton argued for improved wages for nurses, as did the Canadian Congress of Labour. At the same time, some lay people accused nurses of passivity regarding their lack of action in improving their conditions of work.[42] Canadians generally viewed nursing service as indispensable and supported all of its efforts towards professionalization.

The heightened exposure that the war gave nursing also revealed the growing unrest. Their dialogue reflected the ongoing tension that existed among nurses regarding the reality of nursing practice and the ideology of professionalism.[43] Nurses on the home front still worked excessively long hours and under extremely heavy workloads. This contributed to a growing frustration that prompted some nurses to join labour unions. Nursing leaders concluded that the dissatisfaction reported in the local press was simply "destructive criticism" and a reflection of the general turmoil affecting the whole world.[44] The Canadian Nurses Association president warned the membership that if nurses were not prepared to fulfill the expectations of the public, another group would shift them out of the picture.[45] Later, the editor of The Canadian Nurse accused the nurses of being myopic and unable to see beyond their immediate problems. She warned nurses:

> *There are others who will supersede us.* Let us therefore look beyond our immediate field of vision to the unlimited opportunities that await us if we do not allow selfishness, vainglory and shortsightedness to blur the horizon.[46]

Nursing leaders were convinced that if nurses persisted in pursuing the fulfillment of their own wants as opposed to what was expected of them, they would be condemned and nursing as a profession would be doomed. Service, as a key element of nursing, was emphasized time and again but often lost out to the gains available in the trade union movement.[47]

It was clear that the non-nursing unions presented a threat to the national and provincial nursing leadership. Therefore, the professional associations appealed to the membership to support the collective bargaining process that could be undertaken through provincial Labour Relations Committees and further, "to rally to the support of the emerging giantess – the Canadian Nurses Association."[48] Tensions persisted between the vocational wants of the nurses and the growing needs of the public. The nursing leadership was adamant and continued to seek resolution to this dilemma in the ideology of professionalism. The national organization emphasized the fact that the goal of professional nursing was to fulfill the demands of the public and that this concept was to be kept uppermost in the minds of all nurses. Clearly, this idea contradicted the need for adequate financial remuneration promoted in the ideology of the labour movement. For the nursing leaders, to seek more money would have detracted from the idea of noble service, which was essential to their definition of themselves as professionals.

The increasing demand for nurses during the war affected the attitude physicians held towards nurses as well. Throughout the war years, the collaboration between nursing and medicine that occurred on the battlefield also took place on the home front as both professions met the needs of Canadians. Collaboration and consultation became key elements in the relationship between the medical profession and the nursing profession. Suggestions for nursing education continued to be offered by physicians but were less directive in nature and were presented in a more collegial fashion than before.[49] The two professions joined in consultation regarding the expansion of the role of the nurse that would include tasks previously designated to the physician. Up to this point, nurses did not perform certain tasks such as Blood Pressure readings, Subcutaneous injections, Intravenous injections, Intramuscular injections, the taking of blood specimens, or the removal of sutures. After exchanging views, the physicians recommended that nurses "not do these things."[50] Although active intervention on the part of the medical profession was not obvious, physicians continued to limit nursing expertise under the guise of collaboration and consultation.

Similarly, nursing and the society within which it functioned became increasingly involved. This is reflected in the fact that the events that shaped nursing during the war trickled into the popular literature. It was suggested that for every million men in the armed forces, 4,000 nurses were required. Articles and novels were published promoting nursing services in all departments of the military and depicted all nurses as potential heroines. American magazines presented tenth graders as 'sub-debs' who provided nursing care in the home. The wider popular culture emphasized the sacrificial nature of the work while other magazines simply pointed to the importance of certain aspects of nursing, such as public health work. The image of nursing was given a boost by these articles as was the perception that there existed a growing need for nursing services.[51]

Articles in <u>The Canadian Nurse</u> supported the image presented in the popular culture as well when romantic language was used to describe professionalism in nursing. The 'ideal nurse' was a paragon of virtue whose example would overwhelm any potential aspirant to the profession. A professional nurse was intelligent, showed technical skill and good judgment, maintained smooth relationships, carried out whatever the public expected, and was wholesome, attractive, and wise. Supplemental descriptions of professional nursing stated that:

> [It] is the blending of intellectual attainments, attitudes and mental skills based on the principles of scientific medicine and acquired by means of the required training in a school of nursing affiliated with an approved hospital, in conjunction with curative and preventative medicine.[52]

Noble effort, sacrifice and the courage to fight battles were other characteristics of the professional nurse. When all else failed, general staff nursing was promoted in terms of the numerous professional and social opportunities it offered.[53]

Romantic notions associated with nursing were rekindled during World War Two and were supplemented by notions surrounding religious devotion to duty. The war also stimulated poetry such as "Nurses? Curses!":

> Sing us a song of pain and penance --
> Army nurses are all lieutenants.
> Whether they're blondes, brunettes or titans,
> The hell of it is: They have commissions.
> And privates, creatures of low degree,
> Can dream but never hope to be
> More to the nurses than win their hearts
> Than pulses, temperatures and charts.[54]

This poem illustrates the romantic attraction the soldiers had for the nurse who was unavailable as a result of her professional rank. Although it depicts the nurse as a sexual being, she is more interested in her patient as a clinical specimen, not an object of sexual desire. This would suggest that some professional strides had been made.

Romance and religion were joined in the symbol of the nurses cap that truly linked nursing to religion. The war emphasized this link in the term "nursing sister" which was applied to nurses in the Medical Corps and in the veil worn in place of the traditional nurse's cap. Moreover, only unmarried or widowed nurses were accepted for National Service and they had to be childless. Indeed, the Nightingale image persisted in perplexing press reports such as:

> Florence Nightingale, 1944 version, wears khaki battledress and carries her kit on her back. She's sunburned from weeks of pre-invasion training outdoors. These are the type of nurses I met at this hospital as they awaited the order to move overseas; attractive, merry ... kindly, sympathetic ... Pre-embarkation training was no picnic. Day after day they came back to the camp with faces reddened by June sun. They had carried full kit, worn tin helmets for ten or twelve miles. Beside routine marches, the nurses had military drill, and at the end of their training could flash through most difficult manoeuvres like veterans. Camp hygiene, sanitation and purification of water were also in the course for the nurses.[55]

Along with the competency described in this news item, the public demanded that a nurse, or "soldier in white" be morally as pure as her uniform was white.[56] As one student noted:

> If nursing is our Christian duty, then Christ must be our Head. Only in Him can the needs of the community be truly met. Only in Him can those true servants of humanity, the nurses of today, find the spiritual resources necessary for the adequate fulfilling of their daily task.[57]

The continued presence of traditional religious notions suggests that in spite of the advances made towards professionalism, the Nightingale mythology continued to haunt nursing in Canada. As one patient stated:

> We are hard and practical and efficient but one still likes to think that each one of you is obsessed by the same devotion to duty, inspired by the same ideals, and strengthened by the same courage as that heroic woman, Florence Nightingale.[58]

Gender stereotypes prevailed as well. The idea that men ought to be physicians and women ought to be nurses continued to hold sway.[59] Although nursing knowledge was scientific, it was directed toward serving suffering humanity.[60] Press reports from overseas discussed the many hardships encountered by the nursing sisters but always returned to discussion regarding their femininity. Writers repeatedly mentioned the ongoing need nurses had for feminine luxury such as silk stockings and lipstick. It appeared to be important to note that along with her willingness to participate fully in all of the routines associated with medical camp, the nurse was still concerned with packing cosmetics and "fluffy things." All of this evidence would suggest that although competency was important, femininity was to be maintained under all circumstances.

Nonetheless, competent and skilled professional nurses emerged from their wartime experience and on return to Canada their Matron-in-Chief, Agnes Macleod, stated:

> Naturally many returned Nursing Sisters will be taking post-graduate courses, and others will be returning to their former positions ... From time to time it is hoped to improve the conditions under which nurses are asked to work, and it is the desire of this Department to build up a service of which all Canada can be justly proud.[61]

The popular image may have focused on the feminine characteristics of the 'ideal' nurse but nurses themselves flocked to enrol in university educational programs in order to upgrade their professional status in the world of employment.

The war years offered nurses and nursing an opportunity to demonstrate their value to society. Over 4,000 nurses saw active service in the war: two became prisoners of war in Hong Kong and one died as a result of enemy action. This willingness to serve was equalled on the home-front. The success that was realized in this venture was so great that the profession could not meet the growing demand. Difficulties encountered in meeting the demand resulted in investigations into the situation, which were conducted by parties from outside the profession. These inquiries were then followed by major publicity and recruitment campaigns seeking to attract young candidates to nursing. Further government intervention occurred in the form of federal grants to support nursing education. Nursing service was becoming more and more in demand and, at the same time, was gaining more and more respect. This respect kindled expectations by nurses for equitable monetary rewards for their work.

There was little action in this regard during the war but some members of the nursing profession did support ideas that emerged from the labour movement. Although romance, religion and femininity continued to be a part of the nursing package, a clinical role materialized. Taken together, these developments illustrate a continuation of the shift of nursing from a religious vocation to that of a secular profession. Therefore, the years 1939 to 1945 were years in which nurses in Canada worked together both at home and overseas to make nursing skill indispensable to all Canadians and in so doing, placed nursing service firmly within the sphere of professionalism.

CHAPTER FIVE NOTES

[1] Kenneth McNaught, The Pelican History of Canada, (Markham, Ontario: Penguin Books, 1981), p. 269.

[2] Ruth Roach Pierson, "They're Still Women After All": The Second World War and Canadian Womanhood, (Toronto: McClelland & Stewart Inc., 1986), p. 262-263.

[3] Bothwell et al., Canada, 1900-1945, p. 373-375.

[4] J.L.Granatstein, The Ottawa Men: The Civil Service Mandarins, 1935-1957, (Toronto: Oxford University Press, 1982), pp. 274,276.

[5] Doug Owram, The Government Generation, p. 261.

[6] "Grace Fairley to King," CN, Vol. XXXVI, No.1, January 1940, p. 10.

[7] Jean S. Wilson, "The Canadian Red Cross Society War Council," CN, Vol. 35, No.11, November 1939, p. 618.

[8] Ethel Johns, "Let us Take Counsel Together," CN, Vol. XXXVI, No.6, June 1940, pp. 339-341.

[9] "Overseas Mail," CN, Vol. XXXVI, No.3, March 1940, pp. 163.

[10] Ibid., p. 164.

[11] Fanny C. Munroe, "Military Nursing Service," CN, Vol. XXXVI, No.8, August 1940, pp. 482-483.

[12] "Nurses," Mayfair, July, 1943, pp. 74-75.

[13] Videotaped interview with Reta Myers, Halifax, Nova Scotia, 1988. Myers retired from a public health nursing position in Nova Scotia.

[14] Thomas Parran, "Health, Nutrition, and National Defence," CPHJ, Vol. 33, No.3, March 1942, p. 99.

[15] Mildred I. Walker, "Public Health Nursing in Wartime," CN, Vol. 38, No.8, August 1942, pp. 551-552.

[16] Quoted in Gibbon and Mathewson, Three Centuries, p. 457.

[17] If Women Must Work - What of the Children?," CF, May, 1942, pp. 37-38.

[18] "Attention! Two Special Announcements," AARN Annual Reports 1923-1947, 1942,43, p. 5.

[19] Rae Chittick, "An Open Letter To All Members," AARN Annual Reports, 1942-43, p. 3.

[20] "Alberta Association of Registered Nurses - Minutes of Council Meeting, February 7, 1942," AARN Official Minutes, Vol. 5, p. 531.

---

[21] Pearl Stiver, "Nursing: - Past, Present, Future," Canada's Health and Welfare (CHW), Vol. 9, No. 6, pp. 4&5; Dorothy Percy, "Organized Home care," CHW, Vol. 15, No.10, pp. 2&3, Ethel Johns, "The Home Front," CN, Vol. XXXVII, No.9, September 1941, p. 605 and "Thinking for Ourselves," CN, Vol. XXXVI, No.11, November 1940, p. 727.

[22] Kathleen W. Ellis, "Reaction to Publicity," CN, Vol. 39, No.2, February 1943, p. 105.

[23] Kathleen W. Ellis, "The Publicity Campaign," CN, Vol. 38, No.10, October 1942, p. 791.

[24] E.A. Electa MacLennan, "Canada's Nurses at Work," CHW, Vol. 2, No.3, pp. 2&3, Elizabeth Smellie, "Call the V.O.N...," CHW, Vol. 2, No.4, pp. 5&6 and "Head Heart Hand," CHW, Vol. 4, No.10.

[25] "Thinking for Ourselves," CN, Vol. 36, No.11, November 1940, pp. 727-728.

[26] "Making the Front Page," CN, Vol. 39, No.11, November 1943, p. 748.

[27] J.A. Russell, "Making A Comeback," CN, Vol. 39, No.11, November 1943, pp. 737-738.

[28] Muriel A. Ward, "Making Your Choice," CN, Vol. 45, No.6, June 1949, p. 432.

[29] Kathleen W. Ellis, "A Fact Finding Survey," CN. Vol. 39, No.3, March 1943, p. 207, 208.

[30] The Leaf and the Lamp, p. 88.

[31] "Annual Convention of the Alberta Association of Registered Nurses," AARN Official Minutes - Council, Vol.5, p. 471, AARNA.

[32] The Leaf and the Lamp, p. 88, Lyle Creelman, "What of the Future?," CN, Vol. 39, No.1, January 1943, pp. 35-37 and "A Friendly Hearing," CN, Vol. 39, No.6, June 1943, p. 391.

[33] K.W. Ellis, "Report of the General Secretary, 1942-1944," p. 6, CNAA.

[34] Kathleen Russell. "University of Toronto School of Nursing Annual Report," 1941-42, p. 2, B79-004/002, UTA.

[35] "Excerpts from Meeting of the Council, November 27 (?), 1945," in Russell/Tennant Correspondence, A73-0053-006, UTA.

[36] "Proposed Changes in the Preparation for Nursing," CN, Vol.41, No.11, November 1945, pp. 893-894.

[37] Lyle Creelman, "What is Public Health Nursing?," CN, Vol. XXXVII, No.2, February 1941, pp. 111-112.

[38] "Minimum Requirements for Employment in the Field of Public Health Nursing," CN, Vol. 39, no.9, September 1943, pp. 586-588.

[39] "The Public Health Nurse and the Canadian Welfare Council," in The Public Health Nurse (Ottawa:Canadian Welfare Council, 1941), p. 1, MG30, E256, Vol. 21, NAC and Dorothy E. Tate, "Professional Growth in Public Health Nursing Service," CJPH, Vol. 37, No.12, December 1946, pp. 496-499.

[40] Nettie Fidler, "The Preparation for Professional Nursing," ND,(?mid-forties), B79-005/002, File 27, UTA.

[41] The Leaf and the Lamp, pp. 88,89.

[42] C. David Naylor, Private Practice, Public Payment, pp. 122,125 and Mrs. Rex Eaton, "The Lay Woman Looks In," CN, Vol. XXXVI, No.9, September 1940, pp. 565-569.

[43] Marion Lindeburgh, "The President's Address," CN, Vol. 40, No.9, September 1945, p. 616.

[44] M.E. Kerr, "Who Shapes the Future?," CN, Vol. 40, No.11, November 1944, p. 833.

[45] Fanny Munroe, "Facing Facts," CN, Vol. 40, No.10, October 1944, p. 758.

[46] M.E. Kerr, "Unlimited Horizons," CN, Vol. 41, No.8, August 1945, pp. 603,604. Original italics.

[47] Gertrude Hall, "Nursing Care for all People," CN, Vol. 41, No.8, August 1945, p. 618; Fanny Munroe, "The Presidential Address," CN, Vol. 42, No.9, September 1946, p. 736.

[48] M.E. Kerr, "Should We?," CN, Vol. 42, No.11, November 1946, pp. 933-935.

[49] E. Stanley Ryerson, "Physical Activity and Fatigue in Relation to Health: The Value of Physical Education to Nurses," CH, Vol. 18, No.5, May 1941.

[50] Trenholm L. Fisher, "Legal Responsibilities and Privileges," CN, Vol. 41, No.2, February 1945, p. 99.

[51] "Wanted: 55,000 Nurses," LHJ, August, 1942, p. 4, "Meet Ensign Dorothy Weyel," LHJ, January, 1943, pp. 68,69,72,73; Gladys Taber, "Navy Nurse," LHJ, May, 1943, p. 17; "Nurses," Mayfair, July, 1943, pp. 74,75, Betty Hannah Hoffman, "Junior Home Nurses," LHJ, May, 1943, pp. 426-429 and "Medicine and Nursing on the Screen," TNHR, April, 1940, pp. 344-347; Hester James, "A Layman Looks at Public Health," CF, Vol. 21, September, 1941, pp. 179-180.

[52] C. Hopkins, "The Professional Nurse," CN, Vol. 38, No.11, November 1942, pp. 877-878.

[53] Gladys E. Brown, "Have We Kept Our Pledge?," CN, Vol. 39, No.4, April 1943, pp. 277-278 and Rita Curley, "Is General Staff Nursing Worthwhile?," CN, Vol. 39, No.10, October 1943, pp. 675-676.

[54] "Nurses? Curses!," LHJ, September, 1942, p. 4.

[55] Quoted in Gibbon and Mathewson, Three Centuries, p. 469.

[56] Mary McLaughlin, "Religion in the Life of a Nurse," CN, Vol. 42, No.2, February 1946, pp. 158-159; Margaret Angus, "The Public Wants - ," CN, Vol. 51, No.6, June 1955, pp. 444-447.

[57] "The Publicity Campaign," CN, Vol. 38, No.10, October 1942, p. 792.

[58] Edith Wainwright, "A Word from the Patient," Ibid. p. 778.

[59] Franken Meloney, "Women in White," LHJ, March, 1940, p. 11.

[60] Annie W. Goodrich, "The Art of Nursing," TNHR, May, 1940, pp. 434-435.

[61] Quoted in Gibbon and Mathewson, Three Centuries, p. 473.

Chapter Six

NURSING IN POST-WAR CANADA

The immediate post-war period presented nursing with an opportunity to enjoy the achievement of professional status. By this time much of society, including the medical profession, recognized nurses as professionals and valued their expertise. Recognition, however, brought with it additional responsibilities and expectations. The reality of the situation was that the growing demands placed on nursing further underlined the nursing shortage. Medical advances contributed to a growing need for health care services, which created problems for nursing. The problems were rooted in the desperate need for nurses, a need that was exacerbated by the expansion in hospital construction in the post-war era. The growing numbers of nurses who attended the recruitment campaigns contributed to ongoing division within nursing because working conditions remained unsatisfactory and the rank-and-file did not hesitate to complain. Nursing leaders continued to advance the ideology of professionalism but had limited success in an environment that fostered unionism. Although the rank-and-file nurses were much more assertive following their wartime experience, they did make every effort to meet the needs of society. However, their efforts only resulted in frustration, fatigue and confusion. The profession was weakened considerably by these events. Thus the stage was set for a widening gap between the ongoing professional goals of the nursing leadership and the practical demands of the general membership.

Immediately following the war, many nurses agreed "the publicity provided by emergency war service had forced nursing outside its 'splendid isolation' towards a more professional awareness of public service."[1] This awareness was double-edged. The public would now play a significant role in dictating nursing activities while nurses themselves would demand adequate financial compensation for their professional services. Although moderate successes had been realized, new and challenging problems arose within the profession. Interestingly, most of these new problems emanated from nursing's success. That is to say that the clamour for nurses led to heightened expectations in the profession both collectively and individually. When nursing attempted to fulfill these expectations, the profession encountered setbacks that deterred their quest for professionalism.

The most immediate problem concerned the availability of nursing services across Canada. In 1946, the Canadian Nurses Association completed a report on this predicament for the Department of National Health and Welfare. This was a detailed assessment of all levels of nursing services for the years 1943 to 1946. The report concluded that there was an immediate need for 500 nurses in public health and predicted that over the next three years a further 1800 would be required for the development of new programs.[2] Clearly, frustration would be encountered as the government expected more of the nurses to fulfill the demands resulting from the expansion of hospitals. In 1948, the federal government approved $65 million to be spent over the next five years towards hospital construction.

Nurses and hospitals had always had a long association, but in the post-war years, the nature of that association changed. As a group of Ottawa hospital consultants noted:

> [The] public has become more hospital minded and uses hospitals more. More patients are receiving more expensive diagnostic examination and more intensive treatment in a

shorter time ... The hospital is becoming the health center of the community.[3]

Furthermore, the large proportion of acutely ill patients increased the strain and responsibility on the nursing staff so that more nurses and attendants were needed. As patient care responsibilities expanded, the demand for nursing services grew, which, in turn, contributed to a shortage of personnel and an overburdened nursing staff.

Increasing numbers of hospital beds were certainly a part of the problem but poor conditions of work did not make nursing particularly attractive as a career. Improvements needed to be made in order to recruit and retain sufficient numbers of women to the profession. According to Gertrude Hall, Executive Secretary of the Canadian Nurses Association:

It is highly important in the interest of the public that any changes designed not only to improve the method of preparing and utilizing nurses, but also of creating more favourable conditions of service for the latter, should be given whole-hearted endorsation and support by every citizen interested in the health and welfare of the nation.[4]

All groups connected to health care addressed the need to make nursing practice attractive so that women would firstly, enter and secondly, remain for at least "a year or two before commencing their career in marriage and motherhood."[5] These stressful conditions, at least in a small rural hospital were outlined clearly in one matron's observations regarding her work:

I have found out that there are simply not enough hours in a day. As a matron, you have one title but numerous occupations, e.g., housekeeper, x-ray and laboratory technician, operating and case room supervisor, general manager, laundress and cook. At times the matron is the general repair man, armed with screw driver, pair of pliers, and the inevitable bandage scissors, nail file, and bobby pin.

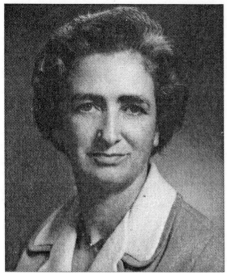

TOP: Alice Girard, CNA President 1958-1960. (Courtesy Helen K. Mussellem Library)

BOTTOM: Sprawling Ottawa Civic Hospital during its sudden expansion after WWII. (Courtesy Ottawa Civic Hospital Archives)

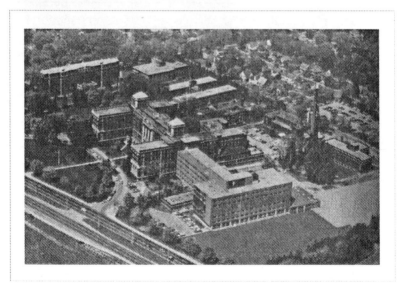

As a buffer for grievances and petty complaints, she attempts to settle staff problems and listens sympathetically to all troubles.[6]

There is not a hint of complaint in this article, but the writer's description illustrates the mounting pressure of responsibilities that faced nurses at the workplace.

There is no doubt that nurses were no longer satisfied with the working conditions with which they had to contend. Those nurses returning from overseas had received educational credits for their military service and took these credits to one of the many expanding university programs offered to them. Their wartime experience both at home and abroad had shown these nurses that their work was valued and further, that they were capable of working independently as they had in battlefield situations. Furthermore, M.E. Kerr, editor of The Canadian Nurse, wrote that they faced the fact that:

Women may believe in the policy of equal pay for equal work but they do little to achieve it. The keynote of ultimate success lies in present day co-operation with other groups having common aims for the betterment of women.[7]

Consequently, by 1945, many nurses had joined a union in order to realize some of these improvements at the workplace.

For the professional associations, union activity was anathema. Union methods did not conform to the dignity, prestige, and high quality of service that was inherent in their professional activity. At the same time, the association reluctantly agreed that unionization was part of the future of nursing. As one observer noted:

The hard fact of the matter is that there are not enough nurses to maintain a minimum health standard in Canada today. Part of the reason for this lies in the fact that the profession at the moment is not sufficiently attractive, and we believe never will be until the nurses themselves as an organized experienced body are prepared to lay down their own conditions of work.[8]

It was very clear that to recruit more women into nursing, the profession would have to be made more attractive. However, rather than address these issues such as better pay and improved working conditions, the nursing leadership relentlessly emphasized service and ignored the union demands supported by many rank-and-file nurses.

The Canadian Nurse published a nine-page article in 1946 entitled "The Professional Status of Nursing" which demonstrated the growing division that existed. The article noted that the priority of the leadership was not in agreement with the membership.[9] In fact, in many respects the leaders promoted past glories of nursing in order to maintain their control over their membership. Nurses were encouraged to bring about a renaissance of the true spirit of nursing. The renaissance was to include the incorporation of manners into nursing behaviour. Rank-and-file demands for democracy in nursing were met with pleas for thoughtfulness, tolerance, and understanding because to follow the path of manners was to follow the "happy" way.[10] Instead of being concerned with salaries, it was more important, the Association agreed, to dress and look the part of the popular conception of the freshly-starched looking individual rushing around doing her bit for the good of humanity because it would make the work of nursing much more interesting.[11] The attitude reflected in this admonition exemplifies the lack of sympathy nursing leaders had for the rank-and-file. Their unwavering focus on their professional vision for nursing had made them resistant to the newly expressed legitimate concerns of the average nurse. Inevitably, this discontent among the rank-and-file grew, causing alienation and division.

The Canadian Nurses Association's quest for a professional identity for nurses had succeeded in this respect. Most Canadians viewed nursing as an essential service. This sentiment, however, was not linked to appropriate financial recognition. Although the collective bargaining process had been approved during the war, it did not fulfill the expectations of the rank-and-file nurses. A non-nurse added more fuel to the fire when she encouraged nurses to: "doubt and to question. You must not blindly accept things as they are, but aim at securing what should be."[12] The growing self-confidence with which nurses emerged from the war presented a fertile state of mind for radical ideas such as these.

Hurting the nurses' cause was "harmful publicity" in the press. According to the Canadian Nurses Association, some journalists portrayed the work life and conditions of nursing in an extremely negative light that was erroneous, misleading, unfair, and adverse. Therefore, the Association resolved to:

> deplore this unfair publicity, inasmuch as those who suffer most by its effects are the sick of the community, and urge all media of publicity to co-operate with hospital boards and management in keeping hospitals staffed and operating under difficult conditions and in gaining for hospitals much needed financial support for construction and operation.[13]

The Canadian Nurses Association acknowledged the existence of division within nursing and concluded that the organizational communication lines needed refurbishing. The nursing leaders decided to improve efforts to inform the rank-and-file of Association activities and also to include them in the decision-making process. The Association also agreed to establish a "Board" or "Joint Committee" in each province to act as a sounding board for the grievances that were currently being aired in the newspapers. Communication was crucial, and the national organization continued to work on "more effective ways of correcting the mistakes of the past and building a stronger, better, and more unified nursing organization."[14]

The Association then expanded these communication efforts to become more closely involved with the federal government. The Canadian Nurses Association recommended to the

Department of National Health and Welfare that a Consultant in nursing be appointed. In 1950, Dorothy Percy began acting in that capacity. Her role was to investigate the shortage of nurses and make recommendations. The professional organization hoped that Percy would be in a position to influence the allocation of funds in order to direct federal funding to educational experiments in nursing. Unfortunately, however, her nursing presence at the Dominion Health Council was minimized. As she noted in a letter to Gertrude Hall, General Secretary of the Canadian Nurses Association:

> I am just beginning to come out from under the three day "sitting marathon" of the Dominion Health Council. (This year the Council members had nice, new, red leather-covered sponge rubber cushioned chairs to sit on. Those of us on "the outer fringe" still had to contend with the old hard chairs. Undemocratic discrimination, I calls it[sic]!).[15]

Percy remained in this position but had limited success in directing funding into nursing education. In fact, federal funds were unavailable to support the Demonstration School of Nursing in Windsor, Ontario that could successfully and economically prepare a skilled clinical nurse in only two years.

Where Percy did have more success was in working with the Dominion Council of Health.[16] She developed a "Film on Recruitment" for them that showed "that nursing can be a satisfying career for young women – and young men – of intelligence and good background."[17] She also acted as a liaison between the provincial and national nursing organizations and the federal government. She maintained a close relationship with the Canadian Nurses Association and was often consulted by the provincial associations. Percy stressed that there existed an "obligation for all nurses to be competent not only in a narrowly professional sense but as citizens, first of their own immediate community, then of their province, their nation, and indeed, of the world."[18] This view reflected her position in the Civil Service of Canada and the patriotic influence that it had on her vision of nursing as a profession.

The rhetoric of the nursing leadership began to combine patriotism with service. One example of this is in the following quote from a contemporary nursing textbook used in Canadian schools of nursing. It described nursing as:

> a service profession whose motives spring from humanitarian impulses ... Being at once womanly and scientific, nursing today is a profession for women who will promote progress in a new civilization based on democratic principles. Preparation for nursing is more than preparation for a professional career; it is preparation for living as an intelligent citizen, as wife and homemaker.[19]

The nursing ideal continued to carry with it romantic notions of service and femininity but now had the additional components of professional science and the duties of citizenry. The combination of these ideas added to the relevancy of nursing and perhaps, gave the career an element of meaningfulness that might attract young women to it in a post-war conservative Canada. Promotions such as these would also add to the mushrooming responsibilities of the nurse which would ultimately contribute to a situation in which the nurse was expected to be 'all things to all people'.

The magnitude of the nursing shortage became acute but the nursing leadership refused to waver from their ideal of the nurse as a powerful individual who "almost alone in our changing society, has maintained work noble; ... has ennobled nursing and raised it to its honoured position."[20] Furthermore, nursing leaders described financial incentives as a "pernicious fallacy." They brought in an expert in industrial management to inform nurses that to improve their "conditions of work" would not necessarily remove their current feelings of dissatisfaction. What was needed, instead, they argued, were psychological incentives such as:

satisfying the longing for encouragement and appreciation; the need for personal achievements as the basis for self-respect and inner security; the opportunity for self-expression; reaching her desired goal of progress and advancement ... This "inner uneasiness" causes nurses to withhold their full cooperation and prevents them from assuming their full share of responsibility for conditions as they exist.[21]

Arguments such as these were meant to suggest that monetary recompense did not bring with it the spiritual and psychological rewards that professionalism would.

Curiously, the shortage of nurses contributed to collaboration and cooperation between the medical profession and nursing. As medicine became more complex, the need for a skilled nurse became more apparent. The relationship had changed as nursing moved from private duty work in the home where nurses were totally dependent on the physician for employment to institutional work where the economic and social arrangement of the hospital work lessened the physician's direct control over the employment of the nurse.[22] Indeed, the nurse often commanded the domain of her ward. Furthermore, "learning to win the nurse's loyalty was part of an intern's initiation and medical lore wryly acknowledged nurses' pivotal roles."[23] Indeed, these post-war years were years in which the medical and nursing professions enjoyed a relationship that approached equality as they participated in the delivery of health care services.

This equality, however, was short-lived and the very fact that nursing service became more and more indispensable created difficulties for some physicians. One confrontation appeared in the pages of the Canadian Medical Association Journal in a debate that addressed the educational preparation of nurses. Two physicians wrote an article entitled, "In Defence of

Nursing" and in their defence of traditional Nightingale nursing they attacked the academic component of nursing programs:

> How would the indefatigable Miss Nightingale, the administrix par excellence, view the growing curriculum with its rising emphasis on academic achievement which is being thrust on "her girls"? ... Miss Nightingale was most preoccupied with the character and personality of nurses ... while her successors seem much more concerned with academic distinction and technical ability ... *We contend that there is only one basic science of nursing and that is simply nursing.*[24]

These physicians viewed a nurse to be a combination of wife, sister and mother rather than an efficient technician, however well intentioned.

Nursing leaders retaliated and presented arguments to justify current educational programs.[25] Others, like Kathleen Russell, demonstrated independence of thought and self-confidence in her response, a reflection of more of the overall growing self-confidence many nurses had attained by the late fifties. She commented on the younger nurse's reaction to the criticisms and wrote:

> Let us hasten to explain that these nurses are relatively youthful. A seasoned old warrior such as the present writer sympathizes with their concern, but suggests that they should not be troubled. The article appears to belong in what might be called true apostolic succession ... Let us be wise enough to let this pass.[26]

Nursing did receive support from colleagues in related professions. Leaders in the social welfare community, such as Charlotte Whitton, joined the discussion. According to her, nursing was "the keystone of the arch supporting the entire structure of the treatment and care of the sick" in the health and healing services.[27] Indeed, as the fundamental link in the health care delivery system, Whitton suggested that:

> There is no profession held, as a whole, in such respect and affection by the people generally, or in whom they place more confidence or to whom they will more readily respond in this time of confusion, concern and search for guidance in a matter so closely touching on their life and weal.[28]

These words reflect the much-improved profile of nursing that was seen by some members of the Canadian public.

Still, many in the profession felt frustrated. Ethel Johns, a former Director of the School of Nursing of the University of British Columbia, expressed the frustration experienced by nurses during her tenure as editor of The Canadian Nurse when she wrote:

> We are not tired of nursing ... We are tired of not being allowed to nurse. We are tired of pinch-hitting for interns, laboratory technicians, orderlies, ward aides, cleaners, and what have you. We are mortally tired of doing other people's work neglecting our own.[29]

Similarly, Kathleen Russell, Director of the School of Nursing at the University of Toronto, recalled the frustration nurses felt when they did not have time to nurse their patients properly:

> We are forced to conclude that this inability to give adequate time to actual nursing, and thus to afford satisfaction to the nurse herself and to her patients, is the main cause of the constant turnover in staff and consequent lack of stability in the nursing service in many hospitals.[30]

Clearly, nursing leaders had not considered how negatively their strategies of over-extension would affect nurses at the workplace.

The constant desire to meet all of the demands articulated by Canadian society simply exhausted the supply. Indeed, by the early fifties, Canadian nurses were leaving Canada to work in the

United States in droves. In one year alone, eight hundred and ten graduate nurses left Canada, and it was feared that their departure would "leave a big gap in the ranks of nursing at a time when Canada has a great demand for nurses to fill both civil and defence needs."[31] The higher U.S. salaries attracted these nurses but the poor working conditions in the average Canadian hospital contributed to their dissatisfaction.

The Canadian Nurses Association realized the "need for a more adequate interpretation of nursing to nurses themselves and to the public who are consumers of nursing service."[32] But even here there were frustrations. Society expected the profession to "adopt high ideals of freedom of action and provide opportunities for growth and economic security for its practitioners."[33] Yet these heightened demands could not be met by a dwindling number of nurses. As Charlotte Whitton perceptively noted:

> The place and responsibility which nursing thus assumes even in the present, but, more so, in the presently emerging health services of the people, throw upon the profession the problem of assuring as wide a variety of specialists, consultants, administrators, and general practitioners as ever confused the senior profession.[34]

Additionally, and perhaps, not surprisingly, the Nightingale legacy lingered on. In the 1950s, one medical historian captured the dilemma facing the profession precisely when he wrote:

> There is no doubt that nursing is moving *toward* professional status, and that it may move further in the future ... Lay nurses have the same right as do those in other vocations to be concerned about adequate income and working conditions, but it would be an unhappy outcome if nurses were to limit their outlook to these considerations. Society expects that nurses like teachers, physicians, and clergyman, will be animated also by a desire to serve. If this spirit is maintained, nursing will continue to be a calling as well as a

vocation; and the rewards of a calling transcend those of a trade.[35]

The old problem of how to reconcile professionalism with the old image of vocation continued to plague nursing even in the post-war period when nurses enjoyed the highest status they ever achieved.

Canadian nurses had fulfilled all of the demands placed on them over the years as a profession, but in so doing created incredible difficulties for themselves. For one thing, their numbers increased significantly. Indeed, between 1932 and 1956, the number of registered nurses trebled. But what they gained in numbers, they lost in homogeneity. This expansion introduced individuals to the profession who came from a variety of backgrounds and included married women as well. Although the leadership remained much the same, the loyalty and commitment of the swelling membership would not be as readily available. Taken together, these developments would contribute to weakening much of the strength, determination, and commitment that had been characteristic of nursing during earlier decades and indeed had brought nursing to its current professional status.

CHAPTER SIX NOTES

[1] Quoted in Linda B. McIntyre, "Towards a Redefinition of Status: Professionalism in Canadian Nursing 1939-1945," p. 89, unpublished MA Thesis, University of Western Ontario, 1984.

[2] "Report on the Nursing Service in Canada," Sept1946, pp.29,41, OCHA.

[3] Neergaard, Agnew, and Craig. "Ottawa Civic Hospital: Summary of Recommendations in the Report," Jan. 5, 1951, p. 1, MG30, E256, NAC.

[4] Gertrude Hall, "The Changing Order and Nursing," p. 11.

[5] "*Obiter Dicta*: What About This Nursing Problem?," CH, Vol.30, No. 6, June 1953, p. 32.

[6] Gleiser, Irene, "The Matron's Point of View," CH, Vol. 31, No.1, January 1954, p. 41.

[7] M.E.K., "Resume of Address on Women in the Post-War World," CN, Vol. 40, No.8, August 1944, p. 553.

[8] "Incentives," CN, Vol. 44, No.11, November 1948, p. 885.

[9] Genevieve Knight Bixler and Roy White Bixler, "The Professional Status of Nursing," CN, Vol. 42, No.1, January 1946, pp. 35-43.

[10] Elizabeth Tweedie, "The Future of Nursing," CN, Vol. 42, No.5, May 1946, pp. 410-411 and "Manners - The Happy Way," CN, Vol. 45, No.11, November 1949, pp. 813-814.

[11] Eileen Mayo, "Canadian Nurses - What of Your Future?," CN, Vol. 42, No.4, April 1946, p. 324.

[12] Dorothy M. Mawdsley, "The Position of Women in the Post-War World," CN, Vol. 40, No.8, August 1944, p. 549.

[13] Gertrude Hall, "CNA Report of the General Secretary," December 5-6, 1947, p. 3, CNAA.

[14] Gertrude Hall, "Talking with a Purpose," CN, Vol. 45, No.1, January 1949, pp. 11-14.

[15] Percy to Hall, April 24, 1950, p. 1, RG29, Vol. 761, 485-5-3, Pt.1, NAC.

[16] "The Council consisted of the Deputy Minister of Pensions and National Health as chairman; the chief medical officer of each province; representatives of labour, farm, and women's groups; and a scientific advisor." See Naylor, p. 98.

[17] Percy Memo to Gilchrist, Director, Information Services, 7-1-50, p. 1, RG29, Vol. 761, 485-5-3, Pt.1, NAC.

[18] Dorothy Percy, "New Occasions," CN, Vol. 49, No.12, Dec.1953, p. 934.

[19] Katherine J. Densford & Millard S. Everett, Ethics for Modern Nurses: Professional Adjustments I, (Philadelphia: W.B.Saunders, 1946), p. iii.

[20] "The Shortage of Nurses," CJPH, Vol. 38, No.11, November 1947, pp. 548-549; Nettie Fidler, "Supply and Demand in Nursing," CJPH, Vol.38, No.11, November 1947, pp. 509-514.

[21] "Incentives," CN, Vol. 44, No.11, November 1948, pp. 885-886.

[22] The Hospitals Act of 1948 had resulted in a boom in hospital construction. According to Agnew "the [hospital] construction grants were of tremendous value in increasing available beds and othe hospital facilities. In the first five years [1948-1953] an additional 46,000 beds were provided and 4,600 new health workers were added to hospital staffs. As a result, the hospital became the centre of the health care program of a particular area and the clinical role of the hospital broadened with the addition of new services and undertakings. Canadian Hospitals, pp. 169,238.

[23] Ellen Condliffe Lagemann, ed., p. 161.

[24] John Zerny and Humphrey Osmond, "In Defence of Nursing," CMAJ, November 1, 1956, Vol. 75, p. 752,753.

[25] Rae Chittick and Moyra Allen, "In Defence of Nursing II," CMAJ, February 1, 1957, Vol. 76, pp. 228-229.

[26] EK Russell, "In Defence of Nursing," CMAJ, Feb. 1957, Vol. 76, p. 244.

[27] Charlotte Whitton, "Address," January 25, 1955, Opening of the Nursing..., MG30, E256, Vol. 52, NAC.

[28] Charlotte Whitton, "Nursing in a Changing Social Structure," 1948, MG30, E256, Vol. 84, NAC.

[29] Quoted in Linda B. McIntyre, "Towards a Redefinition of Status": Professionalism in Canadian Nursing 1939-1945," p. 115.

[30] E. Kathleen Russell, "Fifty Years of Medical Progress," New England Journal of Medicine, Vol.244, no.1, 1951, pp. 439-445.

[31] "Trends in Nursing," CN, Vol. 47, No.12, December 1951, p. 887.

[32] "Minutes - General Meeting, Morning Session," June 28, 1950, Canadian Nurses Association, MG28, I248, Reel M-4605, NAC.

[33] Bixler&Bixler, "The Professional Status,"CN,Vol42,No1, Jan.1946, p43.

[34] Whitton, "The Nurse," CN, Vol.46, No.1, January 1950, p. 25.

[35] Richard H. Shryock, The History of Nursing, (Philadelphia: W.B.Saunders Company, 1959), p. 318. Original italics.

CONCLUSION

Nursing in Canada did not develop in a vacuum but against a backdrop of interrelated activities that held significance for all concerned with health and health services. Canadian nursing began in the nineteenth century as a spiritual vocation rooted in the tradition of Florence Nightingale. As such, the medical profession identified the need for this level of nursing service within the context of a society driven by the need for social and moral reform. The goal of this reform movement was a purified Canada, purified both physically and spiritually. Nurses participated fully in this crusade and became an important resource to both the medical profession and the surrounding society. Over the years this role increased in importance and contributed to the development of an environment within which nurses were given the opportunity to pursue their professional goals. This opportunity was very much involved with the identification of the hospital as the centre for health service delivery and the need for nursing service in that setting.

The attainment of professional status was the driving force behind the actions of the leaders in Canadian nursing and to a varying degree, the general membership of the professional association. At times during periods of societal need, such as wars and epidemic, the professional cause advanced significantly. These events together with actions on the part of nursing leaders, culminated in the attainment of professional status at least by the late forties. Nursing education was standardized and advanced educational programs were available in a number of post-secondary institutions. All provinces demanded a certification test and there was a degree of self-regulation by nursing practitioners. Finally, by the late forties, nursing had become an essential service in that the demand for nurses appeared to be impossible to meet.

The findings of this study demonstrate that nurses in Canada accomplished their goal of shedding the mantle of spiritual vocation that they had worn for decades, and assumed the status of secular professional. Although the path to this victory was erratic at times, the success of nursing was in its willingness to be flexible and to adapt to whatever conditions it faced.

Many factors contributed to this transition. The most important factor was the presence of strong women who took on the leadership of nursing to advance their vision of professionalism. Secondly, the support given them by the rank-and-file membership, although not always unanimous, contributed to the progress made. The intermittent periods of confusion and dissension that existed, stimulated, and often energized progressive activity. The opposition that the medical profession exhibited was a third contributing factor that often functioned favourably. Finally, throughout the twentieth-century, success was directly related to the degree to which nurses themselves were willing to get involved in health care for the betterment of society.

When nursing first appeared on the health care scene in the nineteenth century, it was made up of a group of women who were isolated from the greater society behind the walls of the hospital and the nurses' home. Under the close supervision and training of members of the medical profession, the nurse's only exposure to people was through the medium of illness. Nonetheless, during this time of relative seclusion, strong women worked quietly to organize themselves in such a way as to bring credibility, legitimacy, and eventual independence to their chosen careers.

The First World War and the ensuing flu epidemic presented this semi-organized group of women with an opportunity to serve a society in crisis. Nurses responded enthusiastically and were of invaluable service in helping Canadians face both crises successfully. As a result, society treated them with respect and realized the important role nursing could play in maintaining the health of the community. This was a time during which there existed a considerable amount of interplay between nurses and the community-at-large, a development that was of clear benefit to the realization of nursing's professional aspirations.

Less interaction between nursing and the Canadian public occurred during the twenties because both groups were experiencing post-war disillusionment. Nevertheless, nursing took this opportunity to establish a stronger organizational network. Indeed, three groups of nurses materialized and established themselves as distinct groups within the national association: nursing leaders and educators, public health nurses, and private duty nurses. All three groups participated in an examination of their profession. This self-examination process incorporated suggestions from external sources such as the medical profession and academics. As a result, a determined and committed group of nurses emerged from the twenties with significant gains in terms of their collective self-confidence.

The economic hardships of the thirties created difficulties for everyone. During the Depression, the public complained about the cost of nursing services and the situation was exacerbated by the fact that there appeared to be an over-abundance of unemployed nurses. This circumstance alone set nursing back a few steps, but the publication of the "Weir Report" supported the claim of the nursing leaders that nursing education be upgraded. Nurse educators at the local level took this opportunity to improve nursing education, while rank-and-file nurses worked together to keep both nursing and themselves alive thus bringing considerable recognition to the profession. Nurses received support when their efforts dovetailed with the concerns of their communities, thus adaptability was the key to the continued survival of the profession. The reality of the circumstance was rooted in economics, and nursing survived this predicament with tenacity and determination so that their role in the health of Canadians eventually grew in scope and practice.

The outbreak of World War Two presented nurses with a superb opportunity to become full participants in Canadian society and in so doing, they became indispensable both at home and abroad. The value society ultimately placed on nursing services supported and ensured success for their professional recognition. Clearly, the eventual acknowledgement of professional status for nursing would not have advanced as far as it did without the support of the Canadian public.

Success in the pursuit of professionalism peaked in the post-war period. Nursing had been born in the modern hospital but the post-war expansion in hospital construction contributed to the creation of an excessive demand for nursing service that could not be met. Demands for better salaries and working conditions were not in keeping with the professional ideal and resulted in serious divisions within the profession. The desire to promote their professional ideology blinded the nursing elite to the reality of poor workplace conditions – the primary concern of nursing unions. This major rupture weakened the profession and contributed to disintegration in public support as well.

Furthermore, varying critiques of nursing appeared at all levels of society. Occasionally, individual members of the public accused nurses of passivity in their lack of action at improving their conditions of work.[1] Others believed that nurses owed the community for their very existence and the community had a right to any unique gift or talent they might have.[2] Nurses were also criticized for their apparent indifference to political activity and involvement.[3] As expectations of the profession grew, the public image of the nurse appeared to deteriorate and public relations became a real issue for the nursing associations.

This ambiguity extended to portrayals of the nurse in the popular culture as well. The war had played a major role in promoting the value of nursing service and the resulting nursing shortage only emphasized the need. The expert nurse who was associated with hygienic advice and products elevated the professional image of nursing in the eyes of the public. The situation, however, became confusing for the public and frustrating for nursing because in meeting all of these expectations, the profession had over-extended itself and this only complicated the situation further. In the post-war era, the image of the nurse fluctuated between a devouring and dangerous, albeit necessary, evil and that of a ministering angel of mercy.

NOTES TO CONCLUSION

[1] Mrs. Rex Eaton, "The Lay Woman Looks In," <u>CN</u>, Vol. XXXVI, No.9, September 1940, pp. 565-569.

[2] Edith Wainwright, "A Word From the Patient," <u>CN</u>, Vol. 38, No.10, October 1942, pp. 778-780.

[3] Priscilla Campbell, "Start Talking!," <u>CN</u>, Vol. 43, No.11, November 1947, pp. 844-847.

Afterword

UNIONS, LEADERS AND POLITICIANS: 1960-2000

Since completing my research, receiving my doctorate, and preparing this manuscript for publication, I have reflected on my career in nursing that spans the years not covered in this narrative. I am struck by the fact that a number of themes around leadership that I identified appeared to be ongoing into the latter part of the twentieth-century. One example might be the failure of EP 2000. That is to say that this goal did not become the watershed for the Canadian nursing profession that, perhaps, was anticipated by the nursing leaders in 1982. With that in view, I decided to add an Afterword.

In 1989, the president of the Registered Nurses Association of British Columbia stated, "the future of health care is the future of nursing." This sentiment is an accurate description of Canadian nursing during the last four decades of the twentieth century. As health care ideology moved through the rocky road of socialism to the cutbacks of reform, nursing services were sidelined and the focus of health care became strict fiscal accountability. The success achieved in the fifties became the crisis of the nineties as the role of the nurse took a backseat to the balancing of the budget. As the public became more aware of the crisis, politicians took note and once again, responded as they had during the forties. In 1999, the federal government increased transfer payments to the provinces for health care in the billions of dollars. Furthermore, in this budget, Finance Minister Paul Martin provided an endowment of $25 million to create a NURSE

Fund (Nurses Using Research and Service Evaluation). The Fund is to support a ten-year research program to find solutions to the challenges facing nursing in the next decade. Nursing and health care had become a priority. How did this come about?

I do not propose to summarize the developments in nursing from 1960 to the end of the millennium in a few short pages. I merely want to highlight three important themes that characterized the fate of nursing in the period. The first is the rise of nurses' unions. The second is the crisis in nursing leadership and the third is the difficult political context of health care within which nurses had to work.

While nursing leaders pursued their aspirations of professionalism, regular nurses directed their attention to conditions of work and this led to a significant division between the two groups. This discontinuity in nursing had been an alarming reality for nursing leaders as numbers in the profession grew. Unions emerged across Canada during the seventies that addressed the concerns of the rank-and-file nurses thus gaining their loyalty.[1]

Division, discontent, and frustration described nursing in Canada throughout the seventies and eighties. Division was between the union and the professional association, the Baccalaureate prepared nurse and the Diploma prepared nurse, and even the grassroots maternity nurses and Alberta midwives.[2] Frustration at the workplace was caused by the lack of power nurses experienced within the health care institution bureaucracy. They were told, "nurses are to obey first and grieve later."[3]

The unions offered these nurses a venue and an opportunity to vent their frustration but contributed to some considerable confusion among the rank-and-file as was the case among the striking nurses in British Columbia:

We are striving for professional recognition. However, we cannot achieve the rights, privileges and benefits of professional status without going on strike. But true professionals would not jeopardize their patients by going on strike. So what can we do? Should we give up trying to be professionals? Should we give up ever achieving the wages and working conditions that we know we deserve?[4]

These nurses wondered how they could be committed health care professionals and dedicated union members at the same time. Strikes, however, seemed to provide the answers.

And strike they did, from coast to coast. Indeed, between 1966 and 1982, there were 32 strikes by nurses in Canada.[5] These strikes signalled a new stage in the maturation of nurses' unions and gave nurses a new confidence in determining their socio-economic status and a sense of political efficacy seldom experienced in their professional associations and workplaces. Nursing leaders agreed that strikes were effective but only for a limited time and suggested therefore, that alternatives to strike action should be identified. The strike by Manitoba nurses in 1991 lasted thirty-one days and was one of the longer strikes by any group of nurses in Canada. The nurses walked out on January 1 and the intensity of the strike, in spite of the cold Manitoba winter, contributed to a committed group of nurses who became more assertive and determined not to be trampled.[6]

Through strike-action nurses believed they overcame their humility and gained their self-respect.[7] An added benefit was the camaraderie gained on the picket lines and the education this action gave the public. Indeed, nurses in Brandon, Manitoba commented that, "the strike gave us the opportunity to publicly demonstrate the value we place on being career-oriented professionals who make responsible decisions about patient's lives."[8] The term professional is always present but surrounded in confusion.

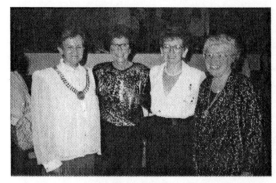

Judith Ritchie wearing the CNA Presidential Chain of Office, Helen Glass, Judith Oulton, and Helen Evans. (Photo courtesy Helen K. Mussellem Library)

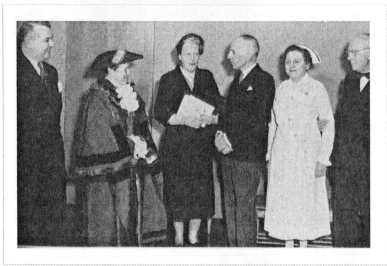

TOP: Charlotte Whitton, Mayor of Ottawa, and Edith G. Young at the opening of the Ottawa Civic Hospital's Education Building. (Courtesy Hospital Archives)

BOTTOM:
Typical image of nurses during a strike.

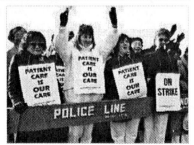

194

The professional associations however, did not support these strikes.[9] Animosity between the unions and the professional associations became quite apparent. In 1987, the United Nurses of Alberta resolved, "UNA is opposed to the position taken by the Professional Association that the minimum standard for Entry to Practice be a Baccalaureate Degree."[10] And, in 1993, this same group called for the resignation of the Alberta Association President, Mary Pat Skene, because of what they argued was a conflict of interest. She was also Vice-President of Caritas, an Edmonton hospital group, but Skene did not resign from either position and the public nature of the debate demonstrates the growing hostility between the two groups. Even the provincial government noted these disputes and expressed concern.[11] On July 16, 1993, a Media Conference brought the two union leaders together with Skene, AARN President, and each gave a brief presentation. The United Nurses of Alberta president focussed on nurses' salaries in relation to the myth that health-care costs were out of control, Skene addressed the need for a long-term plan and the other union leader addressed the difficulties encountered at the workplace.

The ensuing disgruntlement regarding the professional associations stemmed from the fact that while professional fees increased, members perceived they received little in return. The Alberta Association of Registered Nurses increased their registration fee from $140.00 in 1987 to $230.00 (plus GST) in 1996. Union fees, on the other hand, brought salary increases. In a bid to increase commitment to the professional associations, "Special Interest Groups" were set up so that members would participate in their association through their particular clinical practice. The numbers of these "Special Interest Groups," or Associate Members, grew from seven in 1987 to twenty-eight in 1999 but attendance at conventions continued to decline. In fact, in 1995, the Alberta Association of Registered Nurses had to cancel its convention and this, at a time when collegial support was of desperate importance.[12]

Lack of confidence in their professional associations became widely apparent among nurses and was reflected most notably in the fact that executive positions were often uncontested. Indeed, during the mid-nineties, individuals nominated for president-elect in Alberta and Saskatchewan were elected by acclamation and voter turnout for elections averaged around twenty-five percent.[13] The crisis in leadership, however, had begun during a much earlier decade.

By 1956, nursing had enough self-confidence to hold the First Canadian Conference on Nursing and invite representatives from the Canadian Medical Association and the Canadian Hospital Council to discuss the future of nursing. By the end of the fifties, however, nursing faced both a shortage of nurses and also a shortage of leaders. Nursing's strength had been in the unity of the earlier leaders because of their shared cultural values. In 1960, the nursing shortage moved Alice Girard, president of the Canadian Nurses Association, to make the plea, "Wanted Leaders," in her Presidential Address. She wondered whether leaders could be cultivated in the environment of the time.[14] She was not the only one to voice her concern over leadership. Dorothy Percy, Chief Nursing Consultant for the Department of National Health and Welfare, had lamented the lack of leadership in all areas of nursing the previous year.[15] Leadership problems continued to plague nursing throughout the remaining decades of the twentieth-century. The gap between the leaders and the grassroots nurses widened as the leaders continued with their pursuit of professionalization and focus on advanced education.

Throughout the sixties, seventies, and eighties, Canadian nursing leaders consistently strove for increased professional status for the nursing profession. Nursing education had been standardized but the goal became to move nursing programs out of the hospitals and into colleges and universities. In 1982, the Canadian Nurses Association membership adopted the position that "by the year 2000 the minimal educational requirement for entry into the practice of nursing will be successful completion of a baccalaureate degree in nursing."[16] This position, commonly known as "EP 2000" (Entry into Practice):

> was adopted in response to a concern that advances in technology and an increasing emphasis on acute illness and community-based health promotion programs [would] demand a much broader knowledge base ... [for] the delivery of professional nursing care.[17]

The phrase 'EP 2000' was repeated again and again at association meetings of nursing leaders and educators and rationalized in nursing journals.[18] Government funding was necessary to this venture. Governments did give some support to advances in nursing education and the innovative ways of delivering those programs that materialized. The 'EP 2000' drive meant that post-diploma programs were needed for hospital-trained nurses and these programs were created and offered on a part-time or full-time basis so that all Registered Nurses would enrol.[19] This support extended to the establishment of the first Doctoral program in nursing at the University of Alberta, a direct result of collaboration between then Minister of Health, Nancy Betkowski, and the Alberta Association of Registered Nurses.

In spite of these professionalizing strategies and expanding programs, however, the numbers of students entering nursing began to dwindle. Indeed, recruitment and retention became issues of concern.

The problems encountered within the profession involved internal division and confusion, much of which was related to the strategies around 'EP 2000'. Panel presentations at the Canadian Nurses Association convention in 1988 addressed these difficulties. While some individuals noted that nursing might be experiencing a mid-life crisis, one hospital administrator warned "that difficulties within the profession on this issue must be resolved, for it is disconcerting to outsiders to observe fractious factions within."[20] In fact, the gap between staff nurses and nurse administrators moved one nurse to call for staff nurse leaders.[21]

In 1990, 300 participants at a National Nursing Symposium, hosted by the Province of Manitoba, addressed many issues that included, "The Recruitment, Retention and Education of Nurses."[22] Dorothy Pringle, Dean of Nursing at the University of Toronto, concluded that gender bias was at the root of the problem. Nurses were leaving Canada in droves, turf battles were occurring, and this was attributed to pressures within health care and between health care professionals.[23]

Presidents of both provincial and national associations addressed the difficulties encountered by their membership in a similar fashion. Optimistic statements suggesting that the future holds new promise such as, "with a new year come the continuing challenges of nursing. Will we perpetuate alienating behaviours or generate new ways to work toward improving our work and life as nurses?"[24] Indeed, at the close of 1990, Beverley Christensen, a journalist who had a lengthy involvement with the professional nursing associations, published an abbreviated version of a presentation she prepared for the CNA meeting earlier that year. In her article entitled "Just Do It," Christensen exhorted Canadian nurses to make their collective voice heard in the workplace, in the political life of Canada, and everywhere there is power. She, too, commented on the divisions and urged nurses to set aside their differences and learn to support each other instead of shooting inward at each other.[25]

Presidents remained upbeat as Judith Ritchie stated in 1990, "I left Calgary with a real sense that the tide is turning, that momentum for change in a positive direction is building."[26] Incoming CNA president, Fernande Harrison admitted, in 1992, that the need for leadership in nursing was greater that ever.[27] Always promising and optimistic, but empty statements for those nurses being laid off as part of the health care restructuring that was happening at the time. Alberta nurses were hit very hard during this time and their provincial association president counselled them not to focus on the darkness (despair) but to focus on "The Light at the End of the Tunnel"[28] and the picture on the cover of the newsletter was a seagull on a fence with the caption, "Pacing and Worrying." In that same year, 1995, the Federal Minister of Health and Welfare announced that the Principal Nursing Officer position had been eliminated. Clearly, the nursing leadership were out of step with not only their profession but also the world within which they functioned.

This situation was aggravated by the deteriorating image of nursing in the eye of the public as union demands resulted in pictures of striking nurses on picket lines. In fact, nursing was no longer perceived to be the ideal profession for women. In 1986, Working Women magazine named nursing as one of the "dead-end" occupations.[29] The media response always represented a return to the Nightingale legacy. As one writer noted on the editorial page of The Edmonton Journal in 1989:

> If today's nursing "profession" is really interested in regaining the public status which nurses once enjoyed, there's no mystery about how it can be done. As any veteran nurse of the good old days will be happy to tell them: "We got our public respect the old-fashioned way – we earned it ... on the job."[30]

The writer criticized the notion that nurses be baccalaureate-prepared and drew attention to the split between the United Nurses of Alberta and the Alberta Association of Registered Nurses hearkening back to the 'selflessness' of Nightingale.

The image was further complicated by new stories about nurses being charged with killing their patients and during the eighties, for Canadian nurses, the Nelles case jumps to mind. The Canadian Nurse editor-in-chief blamed the media for generating much of the adverse publicity for Susan Nelles and for nursing in its reportage.[31] Charges against Susan Nelles were dropped but the average nurse learned that when trouble comes, support is difficult to find.[32] A deteriorating image would weaken public support and nurses were aware that public opinion greatly influences the goals of the profession, recruitment, the allocation of government resources, and most importantly, the individual nurse's own self-image.[33]

Indeed, this would prove to be the case for nurses in Alberta in 1990. In a province-wide survey of Albertans, funded by the Alberta Association of Registered Nurses, most people (70% - 80%) continued to view the nurse as subservient to the physician, responsible for holding the patient's hand. The authors of this survey concluded:

> The results indicate that nurses have not been successful in portraying a complete and accurate picture of their profession [and that] the public is either not aware of, or ready to accept, the ever expanding role of nursing in the health care system.[34]

Phyllis Giovannetti, a professor in nursing at the University of Alberta, noted that there was a general feeling among staff nurses of losing control and that the current situation would result in alienation and the development of a schism within the profession that was being applauded by other health professionals.[35]

As if the situation within nursing was not serious enough, health-care costs had escalated across Canada to the point that health-care delivery came to be shaped by politicians and finance ministers with an eye to 'the bottom line'. The restructuring of health care that began in the eighties transformed health care delivery from a medical model to a consumer model and this would eventually bring the Canadian public back into the picture. Helen Glass, then president of the Canadian Nurses Association, commented on the implementation of the amended Canada Health Act on July 1, 1984. This Act replaced the previous act of 1983 which "despite all of its positive features perpetuated a very expensive and crisis-orientated system of health care delivery."[36] In order to reduce costs, nurses would play a more significant and autonomous role in the restructuring of the health care system. Events in Alberta under a Conservative government whose goal was to balance the budget exemplify political activities that were occurring in all of the provinces.

In Alberta, nurses participated in the <u>Premier's Commission on Future Health Care for Albertans: The Rainbow Report: Our Vision for Health</u>. Published in 1989, this relatively comprehensive report produced six directions for change and twenty-one recommendations. The focus of the report can be summed up in the catch phrase, "Healthy Albertans living in a healthy Alberta." This would be accomplished through the maintenance of a healthy environment, health education, local health authorities, self-reliant citizens, creation of an ethics centre, and the appointment of a health care advocate.[37] The restructuring would begin as a phased-in approach in 1990 at which time the staffing mix and insured medical services would be examined for cost-effectiveness.

Nurses promoted the concept of 'Primary Health Care' as the most cost-effective delivery of health care services. Nurses would work in the community and the community health centre would be the hub for community health services rather than the hospital.[38] In spite of the AARN's efforts to collaborate with the provincial government to plan the restructuring and accompanying cutbacks, nurses were laid off and the staffing mix in health care institutions changed to include various levels of allied health care workers to rely more heavily on Licensed Practical Nurses, Patient Care Attendants, and Nursing Aides. Indeed, in 1994, the Alberta government completely eliminated funding for nursing research that had been in place since 1981.[39] That same year the AARN reported that "there is no question that as resources become more scarce, there are increasing concerns regarding patient safety, legal aspects of nursing, ethical issues, roles and responsibilities of auxiliary workers, and nurse abuse."[40] The difficulties were rooted in the increased workload and the staffing mix. Multiskilling became the government's solution and nurses were considered replaceable. Multiskilling refers to the proposal that "nursing work, and the work of other health care disciplines, could be generic to a variety of health care workers, and/or that this work could be given to less prepared and less costly individuals."[41]

In 1994, a nursing professor presented a paper to the Alberta Healthcare Association Convention in which she identified some urgent concerns with "Multiskilling the Heath Care Worker." As she concluded:

> In our desire to decrease costs of health care, we have been in a hurry to adopt a strategy such as multiskilling for which there is little positive evidence that it is successful in what it claims to do. It is a quick fix that may make the budget look good in the short term.[42]

Not surprisingly, the "Nurse Replacement Epidemic" stimulated much discussion in the professional journals in columns and in letters to the editor.[43] M.E. Jeans, Executive Director of the Canadian Nurses Association, stated unequivocally, in 1997, that the "CNA does not support or promote multiskilling as a strategy for downsizing." She also noted that she believed the largest threat to the nursing profession was not cutbacks, replacement by others, or increased workloads but "our inability to work together, openly and with trust and understanding toward the common goal of a strengthened nursing profession."[44]

Nurses, unable to find employment, left the country for the financially greener pastures of the United States. The situation was grim. Headlines in the media described the 'burnout' experience of the front-line health care.[45] Hospital closures such as that of the Calgary General Hospital engaged the imagination and interest of all Canadians thus generating considerable public sympathy. The cutbacks were serious as was the public's response.

Alberta Health, in agreement with the Alberta Medical Association made a commitment in 1995-96, "to work together to achieve savings of $100 million by the end of 1997-98."[46] These drastic cutbacks did stimulate some activity among Alberta's nurses. Indeed, the authors of the "Report Card on the Status of Health Reform in Alberta" cautioned the Minister of Health in their recommendations to "revise the government business plan process to make it a more effective instrument in setting direction and strategy."[47] Furthermore, it was the Alberta government's desire to open "The Health Professions Act" that mobilized many nurses to become involved in the activities of their professional association and oppose the passage of Bill 45 in the spring of 1998. The Bill would have eroded self-governance and destroyed mandatory registration, two important responsibilities controlled by the Alberta Association of Registered Nurses.

The events that occurred during the closing decades of the twentieth-century led to a crisis in health care and this crisis resulted in a growing appreciation for the services nurses delivered in the health care system. A survey conducted by the Alberta Association of Registered Nurses demonstrated that Albertans trusted nurses and believed what nurses said, more than physicians, regional health authorities, and politicians. Indeed, according to the pollster, Angus Reid:

> The positive public perception of the nursing profession appears to be a bright spot in Albertans' dim view of the province's ailing health care system ... the public's confidence in the health care system has declined dramatically.[48]

With the image of nursing on the upswing, the Canadian Nurses Association commissioned a study to investigate "The Future Supply of Registered Nurses in Canada" and the results predicted a shortage of up to 113,000 Registered Nurses by the year 2011. The nursing pool had not been renewing itself at a sufficient rate and since 1994, 6,000 graduate nurses had gone to the United

States. Retention and recruitment became subjects for immediate attention.[49] The government responded to one of the major recommendations of the study with the NURSE Fund in February 1999.

As the Executive Director of the Canadian Nurses Association suggested in her article entitled, "The Nineties: Nursing's Decade?," "it's hard to believe the decade could be ours ... try to step back and look at the 'big picture'."[50] Recent events provide some support for this view but it has been a struggle. In spite of the confusion in the nursing profession of the nineties, it has survived and is still looking to 'EP 2000' – now 'EP 2005' – as the culmination of professional status. There is a shortage and recruitment campaigns resemble those of the post-WWII years. This re-birth of nursing in Canada was not a result of the drive for professionalism but was directly related to the public's perceived need of nursing services. Nursing has once again acquired public and political support but not, I would suggest, as a result of the efforts of the nursing leaders but rather, because the practice of nursing is perceived as an integral part of health care service in Canada.

NOTES TO AFTERWORD

[1] "CNA Connection," CN, Sept./86, p.16.
[2] CN, Feb./90, p.22, CN, Aug./90, p.9, AARN Newsletter, Vol. 51, No. 7, p.3.
[3] Jane Wilson, "Why Nurses Leave Nursing," CN, March/87, p.22.
[4] Bernadette Stringer, "Summer of our Discontent," CN, Aug./90, p.18.
[5] Judith Hibberd, "Strikes by Nurses: Part 2," CN, March/92, pp.26-30.
[6] "News," CN, May/91, p.15.
[7] Wendy Armstrong, "Pain, Struggle, Courage," CN, Feb./91, p.14.
[8] Beverley Cumming et al. "The Manitoba Nurses' Strike–Win, Lose or Draw," CN, February, 1992, p.19.
[9] Ibid. Mar./88, p.5.
[10] Ibid. Dec./87, p.2.
[11] Ibid. Dec./88, p.4.
[12] The departure of the Quebec nurses from the Canadian Nurses's Association in 1985, had already weakened the association both structurally and financially.
[13] CN. Sept./89.
[14] Alice Girard. "Wanted Leaders," CN, Vol. 56, No.1, January 1960, pp.17-18.
[15] Dorothy Percy, "Integration and Conservation of Effort in Public Health Nursing," CJPH, Vol. 50, No.3, March 1959, pp.111-116.
[16] "CNA Connection," CN, Feb./88, p.7.
[17] Ibid.
[18] Norma Murray. "Education for Practice," CN, June/88, p.8.
[19] AARN Newsletter, Vol. 45, No. 11, Dec./89, p.4.
[20] "Entry to Practice Enters the Final Stretch," CN, Sept./88, p.16.
[21] Carole Dalton. "The Sleeping Giant Awakes," CN, Oct./90, p.18.
[22] "News," CN, Feb./91, p.11.
[23] Editorials in the Canadian Nurse such as "Success Stories Needed Now!" and articles such as Meryn Stuart, "Nursing: The Endangered Profession," CN, April/93, pp.19-22 indicate the desperate mood of the leaders.
[24] "President's Corner," AARN Newsletter, Feb./89, p.18.
[25] Beverley Christensen. "Just Do It!," CN, Dec./90, p.28. 29.

[26] Judith Ritchie, "Feeling Empowered," CN, Jan./90, p.3.

[27] Fernande Harrison, "Leadership Through Alliances," CN, Sept/92, p.21.

[28] Lillian Douglas, AARN Newsletter, Vol. 51, No. 5, May 1995, p.4,5.

[29] Jane Wilson, CN, Mar./87, p.23.

[30] Olive Elliott, "Nursing needs bolstering: is a university degree enough?," The Edmonton Journal, December, 1989.

[31] Heather Broughton. "A Theory of innocence," CN, Dec./93, p.3.

[32] Jane Wilson. CN, p.22.

[33] Dorothy Robinson-Priest. "The Image of the Nurse," AARN Newsletter, Jan./88, p.20.

[34] Al Turner, Payne, Cook and Associates. "Insight," AARN Newsletter, Mar./90, p.14.

[35] "News," CN, Nov./90, p.12.

[36] Helen Glass. "Editorial: The Nursing Alternative," CN, June/84, p.10.

[37] The Premier's Commission on Future Health Care for Albertans, p.27

[38] Jean Innes. "Health Care Reform Sketching the Future," AARN Newsletter, Sept./87, p.1.

[39] AARN Newsletter,June/94, p.14.

[40] AARN Newsletter, April/94, p.9.

[41] Ibid. January/95, p.7.

[42] Ibid. p.12.

[43] CN, Sept./95, p.13, May/96, p.6, Aug./96, p.8, Jan./97, p.6.

[44] "CNA Connection," CN, Mar./97, p.10.

[45] Maclean's, April 28, 1997, p.24.

[46] Alberta Health. Annual Report, 1995-96, p.6.

[47] Provincial Health Council. Health Checkup, Jan., 1997, Legislature Document.

[48] "Albertans Place Trust in Nurses," AARN Newsletter, Mar./96, p.8.

[49] Barbara Sibbald. "The Future Supply of Registered Nurses in Canada," CN, Jan./98, p.3.

[50] Judith A. Oulton, "Perspective," CN, February 1994, p.9.

Appendix

PRESIDENTS AND LEADERS OF THE CANADIAN NURSES ASSOCIATION[1]

NAME	TERM	POSITION AT TIME OF OFFICE
Mary Agnes Snively	1908-12	Lady Superintendent, Toronto General Hospital
Mary Ard. MacKenzie	1912-14	Chief Superintendent, Victorian Order of Nurses, Ottawa
Sharley P. (Wright)	1914-17	In charge of school of Nursing, New Bryce-Brown Westminster Hospital, BC
Jean I. Gunn	1917-20	Superintendent of Nurses, Toronto General Hospital
Edith MacPherson Dickson	1920-22	Lady Superintendent of Nurses; Assistant Superintendent, Hospital for Consumptives, Weston, Ontario
Jean E. Browne (Thomson)	1922-26	Junior Red Cross Society, Toronto
Flora Madeline Shaw	1926-27	Director, School for Graduate Nurses, McGill University, Montreal

Mabel F. Gray (Acting)	1927-28	Assistant Professor of Nursing, Department of Nursing and Health, University of British Columbia, Vancouver
Mabel F. Hersey	1928-30	Superintendent of Nurses; Director, School of Nursing, Royal Victoria Hospital Montreal
Florence H.M. Emory	1930-34	Assistant Director, School of Nursing, University of Toronto
Ruby M. Simpson	1934-38	Director, Public Health Nursing Service, Saskatchewan Department of Public Health, Regina
Grace M. Fairley	1938-42	Director of Nursing; Principal, School of Nursing, Vancouver General Hospital
Marion Lindeburgh	1942-44	Director and Associate Professor, School of Nursing, McGill University, Montreal
Fanny C. Munroe	1944-46	Superintendent of Nurses; Director, School of Nursing, Royal Victoria Hospital, Montreal
Rae Chittick	1946-48	Associate Professor of Education, University of Alberta, Edmonton
Ethel M. Cryderman	1948-50	Director, Toronto Branch, Victorian Order of Nurses

| Helen G. McArthur | 1950-54 | National Director of Nursing Services, Canadian Red Cross Societies, Toronto |

SNIVELY MEDALS

1936
Mabel Hersey
Jean Gunn
Edith M. Dickson

1938
Jean E. Browne
Jean S. Wilson
Elizabeth Smellie

1940
E.K.Russell
Mother L. Allard
Ethel Johns

1942
Grace Fairley
Eleanor McPhedran
E. Frances Upton

1944
Marion Lindeburgh
Helen L.Randal
Ruby Simpson

HONORARY MEMBERSHIPS

1921
Mary A. Snively

1958
Mother L.Allard
Daisy C. Bridges (ICN)
Edith M. Dickson
Kathleen W. Ellis
Florence Emory
Grace M. Fairley
Mabel Gray
Ethel I. Johns
M. Louise Lyman
Helen L. Randal
E. Kathleen Russell
Ruby M. Simpson
Elizabeth L. Smellie
Jean E. Browne
Jean S. Wilson

EXECUTIVE DIRECTORS OF THE CNA

Jean S. Wilson - 1923-43
Kathleen Ellis - 1943-44
Gertrude Hall - 1944-52
M. Pearl Stiver - 1952-63

EDITORS OF THE CANADIAN NURSE

Helen L. Randal - 1916-24
Jean S. Wilson - 1924-32
Ethel I. Johns - 1932-44
M.E. Kerr - 1944-65

NOTES TO APPENDIX

[1] <u>The Leaf and the Lamp</u>. pp. 75-78. Note the overlap between these lists. This demonstrates the close interrelationships within the elite. These few women spoke for and defined nursing in Canada up to 1950.

SUGGESTIONS FOR FURTHER READING

Barrett, Michele. Women's Oppression Today: The Marxist/Feminist Encounter. New York: Verso, 1990.

Currie, Dawn H. & Valerie Raoul. Anatomy of Gender: Women's Struggle for the Body. Ottawa: Carleton University Press, 1992.

E. Smyth, S. Acker, P. Bourne, A. Prentice (eds.), Challenging Professions: Historical and Contemporary Perspectives on Women's Professional Work. Toronto: University of Toronto Press, 1999.

Dodd, D. and D. Gorham (eds), Caring and Curing: Historical Perspectives on Women and Healing in Canada. Ottawa: University of Ottawa Press, 1994.

Iacovetta, Franca, Mariana Valverde (Eds.). Gender Conflicts: New Essays in Women's History. Toronto: University of Toronto Press, 1992.

Jones, Anne Hudson (Ed.) Images of Nurses: Perspectives from History, Art and Literature. Philadelphia: University of Pennsylvania Press, 1989.

MacPherson, Kathryn. Bedside Matters: The Transformation of Canadian Nursing, 1900-1990. Toronto: Oxford University Press, 1996.

McBryde, Brenda. Quiet Heroines: Nurses of the Second World War. UK: Cakebread Publications, 1989.

McFarland-Icke, Bronwyn Rebekah, Nurses in Nazi Germany: Moral Choice In History. Princeton, NJ: Princeton University Press, 1999.

Nevitt, Joyce. White Caps and Black Bands: Nursing in Newfoundland. Newfoundland: Jesperson Press, 1978.

Riegler, Natalie (Ed.). <u>Nobody Ever Wins a War: The World War I Diaries of Ella Mae Bongard RN</u>. Ottawa: Janeric Enterprises, 1977.

Roberts, Elizabeth. <u>Women's Work 1840-1940</u>. London: MacMillan Education Ltd., 1988.

Scott, Joan Wallach. <u>Gender and the Politics of History</u>. New York: Columbia University Press, 1988.

Smith, Nancy Johnson and Sylvia K. Leduc. <u>Women's Work: Choice, Chance or Socialization</u>? Calgary: Detselig Enterprises, 1992.

The International Nursing History Collective. <u>Nurses of All Nations: A History of the International Council of Nurses- 1899-1999</u>. Philadelphia: Lippincott - Raven Publishers, 1999.

WEB SITES

American Association for the History of Nursing http://www.aahn.org/

AAHN's Nursing History Internet Resources
http://www.aahn.org/weblink.html

An American Nurse at War http://www.nurse-at-war.org/

Archives of Nursing Leadership
http://www.lib.uconn.edu/DoddCenter/ASC/nursing/nursbroc.htm

BC History of Nursing Group http://www3.telus.net/arts/bchn/

The Bellevue Alumnae Center for Nursing History
http://www.foundationnysnurses.org/history.htm

Black Nurses in History
http://www4.umdnj.edu/camlbweb/blacknurses.html

Bonnie and Vern Bullough History of Nursing Collection at the University of Buffalo http://ublib.buffalo.edu/libraries/units/hsl/history/bull.html

Boston University School of Nursing's History of Nursing Archives
http://www.bu.edu/speccol/nursing.htm

Canadian History on the Internet
http://www.ualberta.ca/%7Ebleeck/canada/

The Center for the Study of the History of Nursing
http://www.nursing.upenn.edu/history/

The Florence Nightingale Foundation
http://www.florence-nightingale-foundation.org.uk/

Florence Nightingale Museum
http://www.florence-nightingale.co.uk/

History of the Health Sciences World Wide Web Links
http://www.mla-hhss.org/histlink.htm

Internurse History Page http://www.internurse.com/history/

Margaret M Allemang Centre for the History of Nursing
http://www.allemang.on.ca/

National Archives of Canada http://www.archives.ca/

National Library of Canada Web Service
http://www.nlc-bnc.ca/web/esitemap.htm

Nurses Association of New Brunswick Nursing History Resource Centre
http://www.nanb.nb.ca/en/index1.cfm?access=history0

Nursing History Review (journal)
http://springerjournals.com/store/catalog.html#catnhr

Significant Events in the History of Nursing
http://www4.allencol.edu/%7Esey0/hist1a.html

United Kingdom Centre for the History of Nursing
http://www.qmuc.ac.uk/hn/history/

Zwerdling Nursing Archives http://www.deltiology.com/healthcare.html

INDEX

Alberta Association for Graduate
Nurses, 86, 98
Alberta Association of Registered
Nurses (AARN), iv, 71, 96, 121,
138, 150, 164, 165, 195, 197,
199, 200, 201, 203, 205, 206
Alberta Eugenics Board, 130
Alberta Health, 202, 203, 206
Alberta Provincial Health
Department, 53
Alder Flats, 121
Altruism, 92
American Public Health Association
(APHA), 128
Anglo-Saxon, 35, 87, 88
Attlee, Dr., 113
Baccalaureate, 110, 192, 195
Bedford-Fenwick, Ethel, 36
*Bedside Matters: The Transformation
of Canadian Nursing, 1900-
1990*, 4, 14, 16, 211
Betkowski, Nancy, 197
Biennial Meeting, 136, 144
Brown, Dr. C.P., 16, 131, 140, 167,
207
Browne, Jean E., 40, 74, 75, 136,
138, 207, 209
Bursaries, 154
Calgary Daily Herald, 54
Calgary General Hospital, 52, 62,
82, 137, 202
Calgary Group Nursing Society, 120
'Calling', 15, 40, 98, 99
Cameron, Dr. G. Stewart, 75, 98,
99, 108, 139

Canada At War, 149
Canada Lancet and Practitioner, 90,
118
Canadian Broadcasting Corporation
(CBC), 151
Canadian Congress of Labour, 157
Canadian Forum, The, 109, 136
Canadian Home Journal, 151
Canadian Hospital Council, 95,
112, 196
Canadian Journal of Public Health,
10
Canadian Medical Association
(CMA), 25, 39, 74, 95, 103,
108, 112, 178, 196
*Canadian Medical Association
Journal*, 178
Canadian National Association of
Trained Nurses (CNATN), 2, 36,
46, 58, 62, 64, 71, 78, 84, 98
Canadian National Council of
Women, 44
Canadian Nurse, The, 4, 14, 17, 19,
20, 33, 46, 56, 59, 60, 66, 71,
72, 73, 75, 79, 81, 83, 87, 88,
96, 108, 109, 111, 112, 113,
114, 119, 123, 128, 129, 147,
151, 152, 153, 155, 157, 160,
173, 174, 175, 180, 181, 199,
209
Canadian Nurses Association
(CNA), 1, 2, 4, 14, 17, 39, 40,
72, 74, 78, 83, 86, 87, 98, 109,
112, 114, 121, 137, 144, 151,

154, 156, 157, 158, 170, 171,
    175, 176, 184, 196, 197, 200,
    202, 203, 204, 207
Canadian Press, 151
Canadian Public Health Journal,
    125, 136
Canadian Red Cross, 44, 57, 61, 64,
    75, 76, 78, 144, 164, 209
Canadian War Course, 157
Canadianizing, 88
Caring, 14, 211
Certified Nursing Assistants, 13
Chatelaine, 151
Christian, 26, 30, 161
Class, iv, 17, 40, 136
Cleanliness, 22, 25
Comox, 120, 138
Conflict, 3, 15, 140
Cook, Ramsay, 21, 39, 206
Crimean War, 26
Cryderman, Ethel, 128, 139, 208
Dalhousie University, 16, 54, 77
Department of Health Act, 68
Department of National Health and
    Welfare, 170, 176, 196
Depression, 89, 104, 115, 121, 124,
    125, 134, 137, 141, 142, 187
Diploma Program, 111, 156
Director of Nursing, 46, 72, 82, 98,
    122, 137, 208, 209
Dissension, 82
Division, 16, 63, 92, 192
Dominion Health Council, 57, 66,
    176
Dominion-Provincial Relations,
    113, 114, 137
Dyke, Eunice, 98, 101, 136
Editor, 64, 98, 137
Edmonton Journal, The, 199, 206
Ellis, Kathleen W., 151, 153, 165,
    209
Emergency Nursing Advisor, 151,
    153
EP 2000, 191, 197, 204
Epidemic, 54, 63, 96, 202

Eugenics, 130, 140
Executive Secretary, 71, 137, 171
Family Planning Association, 130
First Canadian Conference on
    Nursing, 196
First World War, 9, 43, 45, 62, 92,
    124, 148, 187, 212
Flu epidemic, 9, 43, 44, 52, 54, 57,
    61, 76, 185, 187
Frustration, 192
Gamp, Sairey, 21
Gender, 16, 162, 211, 212
Gibbon, 45, 62, 63, 98, 164, 167
Glass, Helen, 200, 206
Globe, The, 58, 63, 64
Graduate nurses, 125
Grant, 25, 39
Gunn, Jean, 75, 99, 207, 209
Hall, Gertrude, 39, 62, 63, 166,
    171, 176, 183, 209
Hammill, Ann, 130, 140
Hampton, Isabel, 28, 39
Health, 14, 15, 17, 18, 21, 39, 55,
    57, 63, 72, 78, 88, 96, 97, 99,
    101, 110, 129, 136, 139, 140,
    164, 165, 166, 183, 197, 199,
    200, 201, 203, 205, 206, 208,
    213
Health and Home, 18, 21, 39
Health Professions Act, The, 203
Henry, Edith, 15, 98, 99, 137
Higher Aspect of Nursing, The, 60,
    64
Historiography, 16
Hospital, 15, 18, 22, 30, 31, 32, 34,
    40, 41, 62, 63, 64, 67, 72, 73,
    76, 82, 96, 112, 120, 136, 202,
    207, 208; Closures, 202
Hughes, Linda, 7, 16
Ideology, 15
Image, 206
Immigrants, 129
Influenza epidemic, 43, 52, 53, 54,
    55, 61, 63, 96, 127, 202

Injections: Intramuscular, 159; Intravenous, 159; Subcutaneous, 159

International Council of Nurses (ICN), 36, 41, 79, 89, 97, 99, 209, 212

International Hospital Association, 134

Jeans, M.E., 202

Johns, Ethel, 66, 82, 98, 137, 139, 164, 165, 180, 209

Joint Study Committees, 109

Jones, Agnes Elizabeth, 15, 16, 27, 99, 211

Kaufman, A. R., 130

Kerr, M.E., 14, 166, 173, 209

King George V, 51

Kinnear, Mary, 2, 7, 8, 17, 136

Labour Relations Committee, 157, 158

Lady Stanley Institute for Trained Nurses, The, 81

Leadership, 15, 196, 206, 212

Legitimacy, 96

Liberal, 21

Licensed practical nurses, 13, 201

Lindeburgh, Marion, 97, 111, 112, 137, 139, 166, 208, 209

Livingstone, G.E., 35, 40

MacDougall, Heather, 71, 96, 98

Machin, Miss Mary, 31, 40

Mack, Dr. Theophilus, 30, 40

Mackenzie King, William Lyon, 66, 144

Macleod, Agnes J., 46, 62, 162

MacMurchy, Dr. Helen, 60, 64

Manitoba nurses, 193

Martin, Paul, 191

Massey, The Honourable Vincent, 109, 136

Mathewson, 45, 62, 63, 98, 139, 164, 167

McGill University, 96, 111, 207, 208

McPherson , Kathryn, 4, 14, 15, 16

McWilliams, Margaret, 100, 107, 136

Medical, 15, 18, 51, 75, 89, 99, 101, 110, 112, 139, 148, 149, 153, 161, 169, 184, 203

Melosh, Barbara, 3, 15

Memorial to the Canadian Nurses in the Great War, 66

Metropolitan Life Insurance, 127

Modern Hospital, The, 152

Montreal General Hospital, 22, 25, 30, 35, 39, 40, 91

Multiskilling, 201, 202

Munn, Alice, 72, 96

National Nursing Symposium, 198

National Selective Service, 153

Nelles, Susan, 199

Nightingale, Florence, 5, 17, 20, 25, 26, 27, 28, 29, 30, 31, 34, 35, 37, 39, 40, 61, 73, 124, 125, 133, 139, 161, 162, 179, 181, 185, 199, 213

Notes on Nursing: What it is and What it is Not, 26, 39

Nova Scotia, 54, 58, 76, 121, 164

Nurse educators, 187

NURSE Fund, 192, 204

Nursing: Education, 40, 62, 63, 73, 97; Leaders, 8, 10, 20, 35, 65, 79, 91, 94, 102, 108, 113, 134, 149, 150, 154, 157, 158, 169, 179, 193; Service, 73, 163

Ottawa Civic Hospital, iii, iv, 96, 98, 111, 122, 183

Owram, Doug, 96, 113, 136, 137, 143, 164

Percy, Dorothy, 165, 176, 183, 184, 196, 205

Physician, 15, 16, 137, 140

Pierson, Ruth Roach, 142, 164

Power, 100

Pratt, E.J., 133, 140

Preparation, 53, 89, 99, 147, 165, 166, 177

Principal nursing officer, 199

Pringle, Dorothy, 198
Private duty, 80, 102
Private Duty Committee, 84
Profession, 15, 16, 18, 40, 60, 64,
    97, 99, 139, 205;
    Professionalism, 15, 183, 184;
    Professionalization, 3, 14, 16
*Proposed Curriculum for Schools of
    Nursing in Canada, A*, 112, 137
Provincial associations, 71, 150
Public health, 9, 17, 57, 66, 76, 77,
    85, 102, 126, 127, 129; Nurse,
    16, 55, 79, 97, 128, 139, 166
Public Health Association, 67, 129
Publicity, 165, 167
Pyne, Reginald, 7, 16
Randal, Helen, 71, 72, 96, 209
Rank-and-file, 174
Registered Nurses Association of
    British Columbia (RNABC), 72,
    191
Registration, 58, 71, 96
Registration Act, 58, 71
Religion, 167
Report on Dominion-Provincial
    Relations, 143
Reverby, Susan, 3, 15, 17
Riddell, Reba, 96, 109, 136, 140
Ritchie, Judith, 198, 206
Rockefeller Foundation, 110, 112,
    155
Romance, 161
Ross, Anne E., 40, 46, 49, 50, 51,
    62
Rowell-Sirois Report, 143
Royal Victoria Hospital, 62, 147,
    208
Rural, 15, 79, 97
Russell, Kathleen, 75, 110, 111,
    136, 155, 156, 165, 179, 180,
    184, 209
Ryerson, E. Stanley, 14, 89, 99,
    137, 166
Scottish Nursing Home, 87
Scutari, 26

Shortage, 17, 184
Simpson, Ruby, 112, 127, 137, 139,
    208, 209
Skene, Mary Pat, 195
Smellie, Elizabeth, 79, 85, 97, 98,
    127, 144, 148, 165, 209
Snively, Mary Agnes, 2, 35, 36, 40,
    41, 125, 207, 209
Socialization, 34, 212
Spanish Flu Epidemic, 43
St. Catharine's General Hospital, 30
St. Joseph's, 120
St. Michael's Hospital (Toronto),
    34, 40
St. Thomas, 28, 30
Sterilization, 130, 140
Strikes, 193, 205
Styles, Margaretta, 7, 16
Summer School, 150
Summum Bonum, 45
Superintendent, 31, 35, 52, 73, 91,
    125, 147, 148, 207, 208
*Survey of Nursing Education in
    Canada*, 75, 92, 97, 102, 107,
    136
Sutherland, Neil, 55, 63
Toronto Daily Star, The, 101, 136
Toronto General Hospital, 37, 40,
    41, 61, 75, 76, 94, 125, 207
Toronto School Health Department,
    56
Toronto World, The, 53, 63
Training, 31, 39, 40, 64, 91, 96, 97
Union, 173, 195
United Farm Women's Association,
    54
United Nurses of Alberta (UNA),
    195, 199
United States, 3, 181, 202, 204
University of Manitoba, 45
University of Toronto, iv, 14, 15,
    16, 40, 45, 62, 63, 64, 89, 96,
    110, 136, 155, 165, 180, 198,
    208, 211

Victorian, 20, 25, 28, 37, 55, 63, 78, 128, 152, 207, 208
Victorian Order of Nurses (VON), 55, 63, 78, 128, 148, 152, 207, 208
Volunteers, 53, 63
Wages, 84
Weir Report, The, 75, 102, 134, 187
Weir, George M., 75, 97, 102, 108, 109, 110, 112, 127, 132, 134, 136, 137, 139, 140, 187

Wesley United Church, 130
Whittaker, Jo Ann, 16, 96, 120, 138
Whitton, Charlotte, 157, 179, 181, 184
Wilson, Jean Scantlion, 71, 137, 139, 164, 205, 206, 209
World War II, 9, 10, 11, 142, 148, 164, 211
Young, Sarah Edith, 35, 53, 63, 82, 91, 97, 98, 99, 122, 138

A THOMAS PRESS PUBLICATION

Thomas Press is a publisher of academic titles and works of fiction.

HISTORY
Medieval European, Islamic, Classical, Middle Eastern, Canadian

RELIGION
Comparative Studies, Theology, Mysticism, Islam, Christianity, Judaism

HISTORY IN ART
Byzantine, Islamic, Early Christian

LITERATURE
Literary Criticism, Classics, Ancient Languages, Contemporary Fiction

SOCIAL SCIENCES
Cultural Anthropology, Archaeology, Social Marketing, Political Science

VISIT US ONLINE AT WWW.THOMAS-PRESS.COM

Currently accepting manuscripts.

Printed in the United States
1324800001B/1-63

9 780972 828307